Nerve Conduction and Electromyography for the Physical Therapist

Techniques, Interpretation and Differential Diagnosis

By

Gary Krasilovsky, PT, PhD
Executive Officer
Graduate Center DPT Program
Associate Professor & Director
Hunter College/Graduate Center
DPT Program
New York, New York

Copyright © 2012 Gary Krasilovsky

All rights reserved. No part of this book may be reproduced in any form or by any electronic or mechanical means, including information storage and retrieval systems, without permission in writing from the publisher.

First edition.

ISBN: 978-0615647265

Table of Contents

CHAPTER ONE 1
  Introduction to Electrophysiological Evaluation -
  Peripheral Nerve and Muscle 1

CHAPTER TWO 17
  Instrumentation used in Electroneuromyography
  Examinations 17

CHAPTER THREE 24
  Upper Extremity Motor Nerve Conduction Studies &
  Sensory Nerve Action Potential's (SNAP's) 24
    Motor Nerve Conduction Studies - Overview 24
    Sensory Nerve Conduction Studies 43

CHAPTER FOUR 54
  Lower Extremity Motor Nerve Conduction Studies &
  Sensory Nerve Action Potential's 54
    Motor Nerve Conduction Studies 55
    Sensory Nerve Conduction Studies 62

CHAPTER FIVE 67
  Advanced Techniques of Nerve Studies - Late
  Responses 67
    Somatosensory Evoked Potentials (SSEP's) 67
    Brainstem Auditory Evoked Potentials (BAER's) ... 70
    Visually Evoked Potentials (VEP's) 70
    H- Reflex 71
    F- Wave Testing 73
    Repetitive Nerve Stimulation (RNS) - Myasthenia
    Gravis 74

CHAPTER SIX 79
  Diagnostic Electromyography 79

CHAPTER SEVEN 93
  Problem Solving in Electroneuromyography and Case
  Studies 93
    Case Study # 1: Carpal Tunnel Syndrome 96
    Case Study # 2: Age 5 – Duchenne MD (DMD) 97

Case Study # 3: Suspected L5 Root Compression ... 98
Case Study # 4: Suspected Peripheral Polyneuropathy 100
Case Study #5: EMG Report #1 101
Case Study #6: EMG Report #2 103
Case Study #7: EMG Report #3 104
Case Study #8: Gun Shot Wound to the Cauda Equina, L1 - L2. 106
Case #9: Anterior Glenohumeral Joint Dislocation 108
Case #10: Mid Humeral Fracture 108
Case #11: Multiple Sclerosis 108
Case #12: Isolated Scapula Winging 108
Case #13: Idiopathic Bell's Palsy 108

Appendix A 111
Anatomical Correlates and Associated Impairments 111

Appendix B 113
Common Causes of Peripheral Neuropathies 113

Appendix C 114
Upper Extremity - Root and Peripheral Nerve Innervations 114
Lower Extremity - Root and Peripheral Nerve Innervations 115

References 116

Nerve Conduction Testing and Electromyography for the Physical Therapist: Techniques, Interpretation and Differential Diagnosis

This book is developed to assist physical therapy students and clinicians in learning the techniques, interpretation and use of electroneuromyography evaluation in the differential diagnosis of patients with neuromuscular disorders. It provides the physiological basis and techniques of this diagnostic test through the use of nerve conduction studies and needle electromyography. Readers will learn the application of these techniques to the upper and lower extremities, plus the interpretation of results/reports through case studies. Differential diagnosis of abnormalities that are distributed throughout the neuromuscular system will be presented. Knowledge of basic anatomy related to peripheral nerve and root distributions is being assumed.

Many of the diagrams contained within this book were developed by physical therapists, physicians and others involved in performing electrophysiological testing. This was a collaborative initiative by the National Institute for Occupational Safety and Health of the U. S. Department of Health and Human Services. I have used their publication for many years while teaching this evaluative procedure due to the clarity of the drawings.

This author did not specifically develop the techniques of testing described in this book. This book represents an evolution of teaching electroneuromyography to students in various physical therapy education programs and based upon commonly accepted practices. The specific tests included are an introduction to the most common sites of peripheral nerve testing.

The Guide to Physical Therapist Practice sets a framework of practice patterns for the classification, evaluation, and interventions used by physical therapists in providing services to patients/clients. To assist the reader, the Practice Patterns are highlighted below in which electroneuromyography, also referred to as electrodiagnostic testing or electrophysiological assessment is most significantly indicated:

Preferred Practice Pattern - Musculoskeletal
- Pattern C: Impaired Muscle Performance
- Pattern D: Impaired Joint Mobility, Motor Function, Muscle Performance, and Range of Motion Associated With Connective Tissue Dysfunction
- Pattern F: Impaired Joint Mobility, Motor Function, Muscle Performance, Range of Motion, and Reflex Integrity Associated With Spinal Disorders
- Pattern G: Impaired Joint Mobility, Muscle Performance and Range of Motion Associated with Fracture
- Pattern H: Impaired Joint Mobility, Motor Function, Muscle Performance, and Range of Motion Associated With Joint Arthoplasty

Preferred Practice Pattern - Neuromuscular
- Pattern B: Impaired Neuromotor Development
- Pattern C: Impaired Motor Function and Sensory Integrity Associated with Nonprogressive Disorders of the Central Nervous System-Congenital Origin or Acquired in Infancy or Childhood
- Pattern D: Impaired Motor Function and Sensory Integrity Associated with Nonprogressive Disorders of the Central Nervous System-Acquired in Adolescence or Adulthood

- Pattern F: Impaired Peripheral Nerve Integrity and Muscle Performance Associated with Peripheral Nerve Injury
- Pattern G: Impaired Motor Function and Sensory Integrity Associated with Acute or Chronic Polyneuropathies
- Pattern H: Impaired Motor Function, Peripheral Nerve Integrity, and Sensory Integrity Associated with Nonprogressive Disorders of the Spinal Cord

The author has been a physical therapy clinician, educator, and researcher for almost forty years. His career included advanced training and mentoring in a diagnostic EMG department. Those experiences helped develop an in-depth understanding of how disease affects the peripheral and central nervous system (CNS), and a continued interest in the diagnosis and management of patients with CNS and neuromuscular conditions. This book is also an accumulation of many years of teaching clinical neurology, EMG and nerve conduction testing, and emphasizing the use of this information in differential diagnosis. A key focus of this book is to serve as a review of the differential diagnosis process in neurological physical therapy, and the use of these testing procedures to compliment a thorough and complete physical therapy evaluation. Through understanding the types and implications of abnormal findings revealed in this diagnostic test, the reader will better appreciate when a patient should be referred for an electrodiagnostic evaluation in order to achieve a more accurate diagnosis and optimal therapeutic interventions.

Physical therapists certified by the American Board of Physical Therapy Specialists as Electrophysiologic Certified Specialist (ECS) are exceptionally knowledgeable and skilled in this diagnostic examination. In addition to physical therapists, physicians with specialization in neurology and physiatry are two areas of medicine who are most commonly performing this diagnostic evaluation.

This reference is strictly intended to assist the physical therapist student or clinician in using this information as additional knowledge and to supplement their current understanding of electrophysiological examination. This may also spark an interest in pursuing additional training in this area of specialization, which can best be obtained by contacting the APTA Section on Clinical Electrophysiology and Wound Management.

Objectives:

The reader will be able to:
- Describe the electrophysiological effects of disease processes on peripheral nerve and muscle.
- Perform and interpret a screening neurological evaluation including motor and sensory nerve conduction studies in all four extremities.
- Compare and contrast the normal and abnormal findings of sensory nerve action potentials with motor nerve conduction studies.
- Explain the indications for H-reflex and F-wave testing, somatosensory evoked potentials, brainstem auditory evoked responses, visually evoked potentials and repetitive nerve stimulation and interpret the results of these tests.
- Interpret and explain the various types of waveforms at rest and motor units that may occur during a needle EMG evaluation.
- Explain the proper technique for performing safe and thorough needle electromyography.
- Synthesize results of a complete electroneuromyography examination to determine differential diagnosis, etiology, appropriate intervention

and prognosis. Communicate the results to patients, their family members, and other practitioners.
- Using a hypothetical patient, determine when referral for EMG, nerve conduction studies and advanced techniques may be indicated.

CHAPTER ONE

Introduction to Electrophysiological Evaluation - Peripheral Nerve and Muscle

Upon completion of this chapter, the reader will be able to:
- explain nerve and muscle responses to therapeutic electrical stimulation in healthy individuals and clients with pathology.
- explain and compare the changes in nerve excitability and conductivity secondary to the various classifications of injury.
- explain the basic anatomy and physiology of the peripheral nervous system.

Muscle and Nerve Responses to Neuromuscular Electrical Stimulation

When performing nerve conduction studies, you are using pulsed current stimulation to produce a depolarization waveform in a nerve and then recording over a muscle innervated by that nerve or recording directly over a sensory nerve. You are not using a neuromuscular electrical stimulation device.

Self-assessment quiz. What's your baseline understanding?
1. When stimulating a normal muscle with a therapeutic electrical stimulator, where are the electrodes producing an action potential to evoke a muscle response?
a. Nerve Root
b. Entire peripheral nerve
c. Motor point as it enters the muscle
d. Muscle directly

Answer: You are producing an action potential in the distal segment of the peripheral nerve. This area is referred to as the motor point, where the motor fibers branch out to innervate the muscle fibers.

2. For each of the following patients, will a neuromuscular electrical stimulation unit that uses a short duration current produce a response in a muscle? For the purposes of this self-assessment, assume this patient has no voluntary movement of a limb or specific muscle group.
a. Cerebral Palsy
b. Polio
c. Complete thoracic spinal cord injury (SCI)
d. Spinal Muscular Atrophy
e. Muscular Dystrophy
f. Hemiplegia
g. A partial nerve injury
h. A complete nerve injury

Answers:
a. Cerebral Palsy – the motor unit (MU) is completely intact, so you should obtain a normal muscle (motor) response.
b. Polio – the anterior horn cell (AHC) body is the site of involvement. In severe involvement, the AHC dies due to the infection, and therefore the entire nerve axon degenerates. If all the motor axons to a specific muscle die off, you will not obtain a motor response. You might, however, obtain a response to DC current stimulation if the person had polio within the past year and some muscle fibers are still intact.
c. Complete S. C. I. – this is an injury to the central nervous system (CNS) and therefore you should obtain a normal motor response. If there is severe atrophy, the size of the motor response will be decreased. If a response is absent, there has been an additional lesion affecting the AHC's, which can occur at the level of the injury.
d. Spinal Muscular Atrophy – this is a genetic disorder resulting in AHC death. In muscles severely affected, with

no AHC's remaining intact, you will not obtain a motor response.

e. Muscular Dystrophy – in the later stages of severe involvement, if no viable muscle fiber is intact, you will not obtain a response. In early stages of a myopathy, there are still muscle fibers remaining, and a motor response to stimulation will occur.

f. Hemiplegia – this is a CNS injury and therefore the peripheral nerve and muscle is intact. You will obtain a normal motor response. If there is severe atrophy, the size of the motor response will be decreased. If no response is obtained, there is very high probability of a secondary peripheral nerve lesion.

g. A partial nerve injury – there should be a response if there are adequate motor units (motor axons) remaining. The size of the motor response will depend upon the percentage of motor axons remaining and their proximity to the stimulating electrodes.

h. A complete nerve injury – after 14 days, when Wallerian degeneration has occurred, you will not see a response to stimulation, even if stimulating below the level of the injury. Prior to 14 days, there may be a response to stimulation below the level of the nerve injury.

The clinical testing example described below may be used to evaluate the peripheral nervous system. If a patient who sustained a CVA has a foot-drop, you might assume the foot-drop is due to the CVA. What if the person has recovered good motor function proximally? Nerve compression at the fibula head occurs in many individuals due to prolonged or poor positioning. So, how do you do a quick assessment? Take out a therapeutic electrical stimulator, and try to activate the dorsiflexors (anterior tibialis) or everters (fibularis longus). If you obtain no response on the involved side, but obtain a normal response on the other side (so you know your technique is accurate and the machine works), you can then seek additional testing for nerve compression as the etiology.

Reaction of Degeneration (RD) testing was one method of evaluating the peripheral nervous system prior to the development of diagnostic EMG equipment. It also allows the clinician to evaluate the response of motor units to alternating and pulsatile current stimulation. You must wait 10-14 days after an injury before testing. This will allow for degeneration of the possibly injured nerve to occur.

Electrical Reactions of Muscle and Nerve		
	AC STIMULATION	**DC STIMULATION**
NORMAL R.D. (no RD)	Tetanic Contraction	Brisk twitch
Motor axon is intact and no degeneration has occurred. There may be a neurapraxia.		
PARTIAL R.D.	Diminished response	Diminished response, sluggish contraction
Immediately after an injury before degeneration is complete, or occurs in partial nerve injuries		
FULL R.D.	No response	Slow, sluggish response
Indicates loss of excitability of the muscle. Muscle is denervated		
ABSOLUTE R.D.	No response	No response
Loss of excitability of nerve and muscle. Total connective tissue proliferation		

Figure 1-1 RD Testing: Electrical responses to AC and DC stimulation.

Terminology:
AC Stimulation - alternating current at 100-110 Hz. Phase duration is in the range of 1ms, which is adequate for normally innervated muscle but inadequate in duration to directly depolarize denervated muscle.

DC Stimulation - monophasic current that flows continuously with a pulse duration greater than 10ms. This duration can achieve depolarization of a denervated muscle.

Reaction of Degeneration is normal (no RD) in an upper motor neuron lesion (UMNL). There might be atrophy, but the motor unit should be intact. RD is present in a lower motor neuron lesion (LMNL). There will either be a partial RD finding or a full RD finding, depending upon the severity of the nerve injury. RD is normal in someone with a tendon laceration. There will not be joint movement, but the muscle may still shorten when activated. This is not a typical test, but a clinical example that the nerve is not affected.

Advantages of RD testing
This is a quick, easy way to determine the relative state of innervation of a skeletal muscle with commonly used electrical stimulation equipment. A normal response reveals the superficial fibers of the muscle are innervated. This screening assessment is also non-invasive.

Disadvantages of RD testing
This is a qualitative test unlike other electrodiagnostic tests that provide more quantitative information related to nerve degeneration. Superficial stimulation is insensitive to minor changes in the nerve and muscle. The response may appear normal, since mild nerve involvement will not be observed. This testing can produce a false negative with deep injuries, and can produce a false severe positive with superficial injuries. You can only test superficial muscles with surface

electrical stimulation. If the response does not appear to be normal, you cannot determine the cause of the abnormality.

Electrical Excitability of Nerve and Muscle
This is the foundation for doing nerve conduction studies. You stimulate a nerve proximally above threshold and record distally along that nerve (or the muscle it innervated) to determine the velocity of the action potential (AP) along the nerve and the amplitude of the response.

Transmembrane potential:
The potassium (K+) and calcium (Ca+) ion concentrations cause the potential inside the axon to be -70 to -90 mV compared to outside the nerve membrane. A stimulus of threshold intensity or greater causes the potential inside the axon to increase by approximately 110 mV thus the inside becomes +40 mV higher than outside. This sets up an AP along the entire course of the axon. The intensity of the stimulus must be above threshold to produce an AP. As the intensity is increased, more axons are stimulated.

Propagation of an AP occurs differently in unmyelinated fibers compared to myelinated fibers. Along unmyelinated fibers (Figure 1-2), propagation of an AP is slower because once depolarization is achieved, the AP in one segment produces an AP in the adjacent segment and this process continues along the entire course of a nerve.

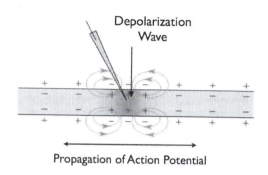

Propagation of Action Potential

Figure 1-2: Action Potential & Propagation along an unmyelinated axon

AP's along a myelinated nerve (Figure 1-3) travel faster since the AP jumps from Node of Ranvier to Node of Ranvier rather than along the anatomical course of the entire axon. The distances between each node varies between 0.2 and 2.0 mm.

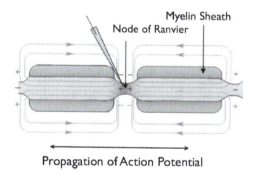

Propagation of Action Potential

Figure 1-3: Action Potential & Propagation along a myelinated nerve axon

The AP travels in both directions along both motor and sensory nerve fibers. The normal direction of flow of an AP is called orthodromic (for sensory this is distal to proximal and for motor this is proximal to distal). The opposite direction of flow of an AP is called antidromic (for sensory this is proximal to distal and for motor fibers this is distal to proximal).

Volume Conduction - Recording an Action Potential
Action potentials travel along the course of a nerve, but also travel beyond the source throughout the body. This is true of any biological potential (EEG, ECG, EMG etc.) While learning to record from nerve or muscle, it is important to understand that you might also be picking up a volume conducted AP's from a nearby nerve or muscle, and not just from the nerve or muscle you are closest to. Recordings of ECG's are a simple example of how cardiac muscle AP's are recorded (without inserting a needle into the heart!). The tissues and body fluids between the (generator) muscle and skin act as volume conductors, which facilitates recording action potentials away from their source.

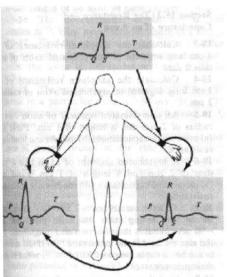

Figure 1-4: Normal Volume Conduction

Implications for Volume Conduction
- What might occur in the UE when stimulating in the upper arm?
- What might occur when trying to record from the Extensor Digitorum Longus with surface electrodes?

Answers:
When performing nerve conduction studies, a target nerve is stimulated at specific sites. If attempting to stimulate the median or ulnar nerve in the medial upper arm, the stimulus might trigger an action potential in more than one nerve if the examiner is not careful on the exact placement of the stimulator and the settings of the stimulator (pulse duration and intensity).

When recording in the forearm as in the extensor digitorum longus (EDL), surface electrodes can easily pick up action potentials generated by the wrist extensors if the subject extends their wrist while trying to activate their EDL. This is an example in kinesiological or biofeedback EMG. Looking at the tracings will not reveal this, but visually observing the movement (if any) will reveal that the tracing might be due to activation of the wrist extensor(s) rather than the target EDL. This is an example of volume conduction. In performing diagnostic EMG, needle electrodes are used and one advantage is they eliminate volume conduction due to their very small radius of picking up action potentials.

Anatomy & Physiology of the Neuromuscular Junction
The diagram in Figure 1-5 displays a normal simplified neuromuscular junction (NMJ) on the left and a NMJ in a patient with Myasthenia Gravis (MG) on the right. The distal segment of the motor nerve (axon terminal) is a primary storage sites for acetylcholine (ACh) contained in synaptic vesicles. The area between the nerve and the receptor field of the muscle is the synaptic cleft. When an

AP reaches the distal segment of the nerve, ACh is released into the synaptic cleft and then binds with the ACh receptors in the muscle. In MG, the number of ACh receptor sites is decreased and their sensitivity to ACh is impaired.

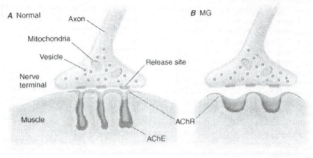

Figure 1-5: The Neuromuscular Junction (A) Normal (B) MG

Electrical Activity at the End Plate
- Miniature end plate potentials (MEPP's). Sub threshold release of ACh, which occurs constantly in a healthy individual.
- Synaptic Vesicles contain ten thousand quanta of ACh on the axon terminal.
- When EPP's exceed threshold, an action potential is generated, resulting in a graded response that increases proportionally to the release of ACh.

Muscle Contraction
- ACh crosses the synaptic cleft of the NMJ and bonds with postsynaptic receptor sites.
- ACh reacts with receptor sites.
- Muscle sarcolemmas depolarize and this spreads throughout the transverse tubular system and triggers the sacroplasmic reticulum to release calcium and begin a mechanical muscle contraction.
- Relaxation occurs after 5-10 msec. with uptake of calcium back into storage sites.

Classifications of Nerve Injuries

Seddon is well known for describing the three degrees of a peripheral nerve lesion. In order from mild to most severe, these include neuropraxia, axonotmesis and neurotmesis. Sunderland expanded upon neurotmesis to include three subdivisions of severity of this most serious type of peripheral nerve injury. Sunderland's subdivisions of neurotmesis provide better grading of the changes to the internal sheaths within a peripheral nerve, which compartmentalize the axon bundles into fascicles.

Neurapraxia (Type I)- Blockage of conduction without loss of continuity of the nerve axon. This usually reverses spontaneously with immediate release of compression (ex: sitting with legs crossed and one leg "falls asleep"). If the duration of compression is prolonged, recovery from conduction block could take weeks.

Axonotomesis (Type II)- Damage to the axon with subsequent Wallerian Degeneration. Connective tissue sheaths and basement membrane of the nerve axon remains intact. Conduction ends immediately. Regeneration occurs at 1-2mm/day and is usually effective unless the lesion is very proximal in long nerve segments.

Neurotmesis

Type III: Damage to the axon and endoneurium but with preservation of the perineurium and fascicular arrangement. Regeneration is less complete but with functional recovery. Changes of the internal architecture of the nerve and connective tissue proliferation, which worsens in type IV & V, will greatly affect recovery, even with surgical repair.
Type IV: Damage to the axon, endoneurium and perineurium, although the nerve remains visually intact. Regeneration is poorly oriented and less effective.

Type V: Complete anatomical transection of the nerve. Regeneration is poor, due to many factors including time of surgical repair and internal scarring.

Factors Affecting Nerve Physiology
There are many pathological and physiological factors that affect nerve conduction results and interpretation of these results. The physiological basis and diagnostic interpretation of all these factors is beyond the scope of this introductory reference. (See reference list for more sources). Described below are some of the major factors affecting results and interpretation of nerve conduction studies.

- **Conduction Block**: Failure of an AP in one or more nerve axons to continue beyond a specific point in the neuraxis. Conduction block is often due to localized compression (neurapraxia). The nerve axon(s) conduct normally above or below the level of compression, but not through the site of compression. To confirm a conduction block, when stimulating and recording distal to the block, the compound muscle action potential (CMAP) amplitude will be a minimum of 20% greater compared to the CMAP elicited when stimulating proximal to the conduction block.
- **Temporal Dispersion (TD)**: Refers to the increased duration of a nerve action potential or CMAP. When stimulating and recording over long nerve segments, the AP's of slow conducting fibers increasingly lag behind the AP's of fast conducting fibers. This results in the duration of the proximal compound nerve action potential (NAP) to increase at least 20% compared to the distal NAP. The NAP also decreases in amplitude over these longer distances, which occurs due to phase cancellation within the NAP. In combination, this results in the area under the curve of the compound NAP to be decreased in the proximal NAP (for example in axilla to the second digit) compared to the distal NAP (wrist to

second digit). Temporal dispersion does not normally occur in CMAP long distances. In performing motor nerve conduction studies, if TD of the CMAP is revealed, this is often associated with conduction block or demyelination between the proximal and distal stimulation sites. For example, in Guillian Barre' Syndrome or ulnar nerve compression at the elbow, the CMAP will reveal TD.
- **CMAP and SNAP amplitude changes:** The amplitudes of CMAP should not change when stimulating proximally or distally and recording distally. The amplitude of SNAP's does normally decrease as the distance between the stimulation and recording sites increases, as described above in TD.
- **Limb temperature** affects nerve conduction velocity and therefore must be measured and the muscle/limb warmed if necessary. The skin temperature of the upper extremity should be at 91 degrees and the lower extremity should be 88 degrees. A cold limb will decrease conduction velocity and a warmed limb (as in after exercise) will slightly increase CV. If necessary, the extremity to be tested should be warmed first. Heating modalities such as infrared heat lamp can be used to warm a cold extremity. Excess warming of an extremity (107 degrees) will increase CV but decrease amplitude by up to 50 percent.

Severity of Peripheral Neuropathies
- **Mild demyelination:** Delayed conduction of the sensory greater than motor fibers. There may be decreased amplitude of the response due to partial conduction block. Distal latencies may be prolonged. Temporal dispersion may be present.
- **Advanced demyelination:** More severe slowing of conduction in sensory and motor fibers with associated increased temporal dispersion and conduction block

(which also results in decreased amplitude of the evoked responses).
- **Axonal loss without demyelination:** SNAP's decreased in amplitude or absent. CMAP amplitude is proportionally decreased. Motor conduction velocity (MCV) is normal or only slightly decreased.
- **Axonal loss with demyelination:** Considerable delay in conduction and greater temporal dispersion of the evoked responses. Amplitudes will be decreased.
- Total Axonal Degeneration: No conduction occurs.

Categories and Etiologies of Peripheral Nerve Lesions
- Mononeuropathy - One nerve is affected, usually due to compression or traction.
- Mononeuropathy multiplex - multiple peripheral nerves become affected over time. Discrete lesions of individual peripheral nerves. Often vascular in origin.
- Polyneuropathy - Multiple nerves affected due to systemic disease or drug/chemical toxicity. Examples include Guillian Barre' Syndrome, Lyme disease, Diabetes, Alcohol Abuse or chemotherapy. Often described as presenting with complaints in a glove and stocking distribution.
- Radiculopathy - one or more spinal roots involved. Etiology includes disc herniation, foramen encroachment, tumor, and Herpes Zoster infection.

Significance of Nerve Abnormalities
- Sensory disturbances occur before motor deficits.
- Location and pattern of abnormalities helps determine the type of peripheral neuropathy and possible etiology.

Significance of Neuromuscular Junction Abnormalities
The most common disorder affecting the neuromuscular junction (NMJ) is Myasthenia Gravis. Clients with this disorder may present with fatigue that worsens as the day

progresses and begins to resolve after rest. This disorder affects the amount of ACh stored at the proximal end of the NM junction and a reduction in the number and availability of receptor sites on the muscle side of the NMJ. Botulism poisoning also affects the NMJ. Honey that is poorly prepared in the canning process can contain botulism spores. Infants should not be given honey under one year of age due to the risk factors. Botox, used in the management of spasticity, blocks the NMJ. Testing for this disorder will be covered in Chapter Five.

Electrophysiological basis for diagnostic EMG
The electrical characteristic of each MU is based upon the number of muscle fibers innervated by each motor nerve axon. This ratio of one axon to the number of muscle fibers is the innervation ratio. Extra-ocular muscles may only have five muscle fibers per MU, while intrinsic hand muscles may have an innervation ratio of 1:100 and the gastrocnemius ratio is 1:2,000. The configuration of the summated (compound) motor unit action potential (CMAP) will change in different disease processes. Diagnostic EMG reveals these changes and assists in the diagnosis. When using needle electrodes, the recording electrode is placed within the skeletal muscle generating the AP. The waveform of the recorded motor unit action potential varies with the location of the recording tip relative to the source of the motor unit potential. The closer the tip of the needle to the firing motor unit, the larger and more accurate the configuration of that MU. Therefore, the same MU shows multiple profiles depending on the site of the exploring needle in relation to each MU. The recording needle electrode is used to sample many areas within the muscle to visualize those MU's closest to the tip of the needle to best visualize their true electrical configuration. Abnormal electrical potentials discharged at rest can be identified during needle EMG, and will add to the

diagnostic picture. Needle EMG will be described in detail in chapter six.

Nerve Conduction Studies record the CMAP or sensory nerve action potential (SNAP) and allow evaluation of the conduction velocity and amplitude of each nerve tested. The most common variables that affect nerve conduction velocity are demyelination or compression.

In combination, nerve conduction studies and diagnostic EMG gives data on the anatomical and physiological status of each peripheral nerve, information on the status of the total compliment of intact nerve axons via amplitude of the response and specific detailed information on the status of individual MU's. This combination of information, coupled with a complete history and clinical evaluation provides excellent information that can lead to an accurate diagnosis of a disease process affecting the peripheral neuromuscular system.

CHAPTER TWO

Instrumentation used in Electroneuromyography Examinations

Upon completion of this chapter, the reader will be able to:
- compare and contrast the use of surface electrodes and needle electrodes used in electroneuromyography.
- describe the selection of recording or stimulating electrodes in different testing protocols.
- describe a differential amplifier and its significance in nerve conduction testing and diagnostic EMG.
- avoid electrical artifact (noise) during recording of biological signals.

Surface electrodes (Figure 2-1) are used in recording biological signals generated within the body. They are used in performing electrocardiograms, EMG biofeedback, and nerve conduction studies. The type of surface electrode used varies depending upon the recording site and the type of action potential being measured. They cannot be used as the active recording electrode in diagnostic electromyography. Round, surface disc electrodes are typically used for MCV, orthodromic SNAP's, or other direct nerve-to-nerve recordings. They are applied to the skin with tape or self-adhesive collars. Types of electrodes:
- Round, flat silver silver-chloride discs 1-2 cm in diameter. Most durable and easy to clean and reuse.
- Ground electrode – serves to reduce artifact. Round bare metal with wire attached. Larger than the active and reference electrodes.
- Disposable self-adhesive electrodes (2 types shown).
- Block electrode – two round disc electrodes embedded in a plastic bar, which standardizes distance between both

active & reference electrodes. Can be used to record or stimulate over nerve.
- Stainless steel ring electrodes used for SNAP's

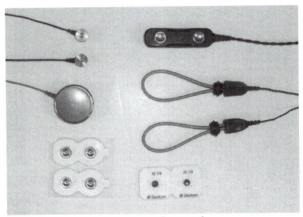

Figure 2-1: Surface recording electrodes

EMG Electrode	Features	
Monopolar	0.4 mm diameter. Single shaft needle with shaft insulated. Exposed tip is recording surface. Second reference electrode and ground electrode required.	Requires second surface or needle electrode as a reference. Easy insertion, less painful than concentric needle. Low impedance.
Concentric (Coaxial)	0.1 mm diameter wire inside #26 hypodermic needle. Shaft of needle is reference electrode, and wire inside is active electrode.	Very localized area of recording. No additional reference electrode required.
Bipolar (Dual Coaxial)	Two 0.1 mm diameter wires inside a #23 hypodermic needle. Shaft of needle is the ground. Two wires are the active and reference electrodes.	No additional ground or reference electrode required. Very localized recording area.
Flexible Wire Electrode	Used in pairs. Inserted using a cannula (hypodermic needle). Used in kinesiological EMG	Insulated, except at the tip of the electrode. Flexible, will not break. Used in kinesiological EMG.

Figure 2-2: EMG needle electrodes and features.

Needles electrodes (see Figure 2-2) vary in configuration depending upon the need for specific recording of motor unit action potentials. Needle electrodes must be used during diagnostic electromyography.

Monopolar needle electrodes are very small diameter; vary in lengths including 12 mm EEG needles (also used for SSEP's), 25mm, 37mm, 50mm and 75mm. The entire shaft of the needle is coated in Teflon® or other substances to insulate and reduce friction. Only the tip of the electrode is bare and serves as the recording area of the electrode. They are less painful than larger diameter needles. This is the needle of choice for many EMG tests. They are single use (per patient) and then discarded.

Concentric needle electrodes use a typical hypodermic needle with an insulated wire within. The shaft of the external needle serves as the reference electrode and the tip of the centrally located wire serves as the active electrode. Their recording area is very localized and they are more accurate in recording EMG potentials. However, they are more painful due to the larger diameter of the needle.

Bipolar needle electrode uses a slightly larger diameter hypodermic needle than the concentric needle. This electrode has two separately insulated wires within, which act as the active and reference electrodes, while the shaft of this needle serves as the ground. This is used more exclusively for evaluating individual muscle fibers and not typically for standard diagnostic testing. Bipolar and concentric needle electrodes can be sterilized and reused, which requires careful examination of the tip to ensure no burrs or dulling has occurred before reuse.

Flexible wire electrodes are used in kinesiological EMG studies. They are inserted into a muscle via a regular hypodermic needle. The insertion needle is withdrawn and the flexible wire remains in place within the muscle during kinesiological evaluations.

Advantages and Disadvantages of Surface Recording Electrodes
- Advantages
  - Easy to obtain
  - Easy to apply to the skin
  - Non-invasive → easy to obtain patient consent
- Disadvantages
  - General pickup area
  - Non-specific for one muscle
  - Can only use on superficial muscles
  - High possibility of movement artifact
  - Cannot be the only electrode used in diagnostic EMG.

Advantages and Disadvantages of Needle Recording Electrodes
- Advantages
  - Very specific recording within one muscle
  - Necessary for diagnostic EMG
  - Eliminates disadvantages of surface electrodes.
- Disadvantages
  - Invasive for non-diagnostic studies
  - Painful for the patient
  - Risk of infection
  - Risk of hitting a nerve or blood vessel.
  - Risk of pneumothorax during EMG of serratus or intercostal muscles.
  - Harder to get patient consent for research
  - Records from a small area within the muscle

Amplifier & settings
The biological signals being recorded throughout this testing are very small. They must be greatly amplified to be visualized and measured. A clinician cannot take any amplifier to achieve visualization of these potentials. Generalized amplification would result in amplifying electrical noise that would greatly interfere with visualizing the biological signal. Therefore, a specialized differential amplifier is required. This specialized device amplifies the electrical difference occurring between the two (active and reference) recording electrodes, providing a clean and easily recognized electrical signal that can then be measured and evaluated. The amplifier rejects random electrical noise or artifact that occurs equally under both electrodes. This is called common mode rejection. The amplifier has three input plugs. The active electrode is typically plugged into the negative-up jack, the reference electrode is plugged into the positive down jack, and the ground electrode is placed into the jack specifically labeled for the ground electrode. EMG convention was determined to include that negative is an upward deflection of the action potential and positive is a downward deflection.

Electroneuromyography equipment is typically computer based. Menus are available for selecting the specific type of testing to be performed. Based upon whether the next test will be a motor conduction study, sensory nerve test, diagnostic EMG, or other specific test, the parameters of the amplifier are all pre-selected. This includes the amount of amplification of the signal, the time base(sweep speed) of the visual display across the computer screen, and settings (filters) on the amplifier to eliminate or reduce electrical artifact while preserving the true biological signal. Additional specific information on EMG equipment and settings are readily available from any commercial vendor of electroneuromyography equipment. No, you can't build one yourself from an old stereo. Examples of typical settings for performing NCV's and EMG are described below. The screen (or oscilloscope) has vertical divisions (to assist in measuring amplitude) and horizontal divisions (to assist in measuring latency or overall duration).

- Sensitivity/gain/amplification settings
    - SNAPs - 10 uV to 20uV/division.
    - MCVs - 2000uV (2mV)/division.
    - EMG - 100uV to 200uV for most pathological waveforms at rest and/or motor units to be well displayed visually. One microvolt (uV) is equal to one millionth of a volt.
- Sweep Speed (time base) – 1ms to 5ms/division for conduction studies, with each sweep triggered by each pulsed electrical stimulation once/second. During EMG studies, 10 ms/division with the visual display revealing a time period of 100ms and displaying continuously.
- Filter settings/Frequency Response
    - 10 Hz to 10,000 Hz
    - Filters out electrical activity outside these ranges
    - Accurately responds and displays AP's that change configuration very rapidly. For example, fibrillation potentials are signals that change configuration in 1-2ms. If the responsiveness of the amplifier (frequency response) is to low, the fibrillation potential will appear distorted.

Artifacts to Recording EMG
- Electrode Noise – Disc electrodes must be clean!
- Amplifier Noise – If baseline is thick, check gain setting and high frequency filter setting being too high
- Equipment Problems – defective electrodes, wires broken within insulation (not visible). Poor grounding.
- Movement artifact – electrodes or their wires moving on the skin during limb movement.

- Electrostatic & Electromagnetic Waves – Motors, other equipment on same electrical circuit can be problematic.

Reducing Artifact
- Be sure all pairs of electrodes are same size and condition.
- Use short, well-shielded electrode cables. If possible, use telemetry system (for kinesiological EMG).
- Properly ground patient, bed, everything touching patient and/or examiner.
- Use a 50-60 Hz filter.
- EMG unit should be on an isolated electrical current.

CHAPTER THREE

Upper Extremity Motor Nerve Conduction Studies & Sensory Nerve Action Potential's (SNAP's)

Upon completion of this chapter, the reader will:
- be able to explain the rationale for performing motor nerve and sensory nerve conduction testing of peripheral nerves of the upper extremity (UE).
- be able explain the selection of the most appropriate tests of the UE based upon the potential diagnosis of the patient.
- be able to describe and explain the technique for performing motor and sensory nerve conduction studies on the median, ulnar and radial nerves.
- be able to interpret the results of these tests based upon normal values to assist in the eventual diagnosis of the patient.
- determine the location of a peripheral nerve lesion, estimate the extent of this lesion, and determine the need for additional nerve conduction studies and EMG.

Motor Nerve Conduction Studies - Overview
- Tests the integrity of the peripheral nerve
- Demyelination slows conduction velocity
- Localized compression reduces amplitude &/or conduction velocity at the site of compression. Conduction velocity (CV) in nerve segments above or below localized compression is normal in a neurapraxia.
- Conduction velocity reveals velocity of fastest conducting fibers. Amplitude reveals relative percentage of fibers conducting.
- A significant number of fibers must be demyelinated or blocked to reveal an abnormal conduction velocity.
- Mild involvement may appear to be WNL's.

Motor and sensory nerve conduction studies are performed using equipment that is specifically designed for this testing. In motor nerve conduction studies, recording electrodes are placed over a distal innervated muscle of the nerve to be tested. This helps in testing the most distal segment of the nerve, which is where most pathological conditions begin to damage the nerve axon. The nerve is then stimulated to produce an action potential, which travels in both directions along the nerve fibers. When performing motor conduction studies, the nerve action potential reaches the neuromuscular junction, resulting in the release of ACh, which crosses the synaptic cleft and bonds with the receptor sites in the muscle causing depolarization of the muscle. For motor conduction studies, the main focus is on measuring the resultant compound muscle action potential (CMAP) as the muscle contraction occurs. The sites of stimulation will be explained for each of the most common UE nerves tested (median, ulnar and radial).

Stimulator and Stimulation Technique
The stimulator uses a monophasic pulsed current with a cathode (negative) and anode (positive) prong. The settings are preset with modern computer based EMG machines, with typical frequency of one per second; pulse duration of .05 or .1ms duration. The cathode is always placed closest to the active electrode in order to produce the best action potential. Stimulating with the anode electrode can produce an anode block of the AP travelling in the desired direction.

Supramaximal stimulation - When performing nerve conduction studies, the intensity of nerve stimulation is "supramaximal". Supramaximal stimulation is reached when the amplitude or latency of the measured response no longer improves as the intensity of stimulation has been increased. This means that all axons are being depolarized with the stimulation and if the intensity is turned up more, no additional fibers are depolarized. This is important to be sure all intact fibers are responding so the measurement is a true reflection of the optimal function of the peripheral nerve.

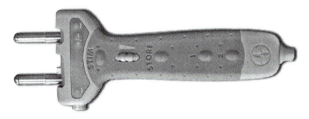

Figure 3-1: Nerve stimulator used in performing NCV's. Photograph used with permission: Cadwell Laboratories, Inc.

Placement of Electrodes and Measurement
Three electrodes are used. The active electrode is placed over the belly of the muscle. A reference electrode is placed distally over the tendon of the same muscle. A third, ground electrode, is placed between the stimulator and the active electrode. Conductive gel is used between each electrode and the skin to improve recording of the AP and is also used on each tip of the stimulator. When stimulating a motor nerve, a compound muscle action potential (CMAP) is produced. In some displays, the first component of this display is the stimulus artifact. This is a break or vertical deflection in the waveform that the machine displays to allow the clinician to measure, in time, when the stimulus was delivered to the nerve being tested. In most computer displays, the tracing begins at the time of nerve stimulation. The time from the stimulus artifact to the beginning of the CMAP (takeoff point) is the latency (see Figure 3-2). This is the time, in milliseconds (ms), it took for the AP to travel from the cathode of the stimulator to the end of the motor axon, cause release of ACh, and produce the depolarization of the muscle membranes and resultant muscle contraction.

The time delay in this process is one reason the distal latencies are interpreted differently than conduction velocity along a pure nerve segment. The initial deflection is produced by the muscle fibers that are innervated by the fastest conducting motor nerve axons. Unless the entire fast conducting, myelinated axons are involved in a pathological process, the latency will be normal.

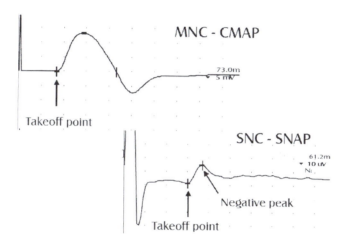

Figure 3-2: Latency of motor conduction testing (top) and sensory nerve action potential (SNAP) (bottom). Photograph used with permission: Cadwell Laboratories, Inc.

The amplitude of the response (see Figure 3-3) is also measured and indicates the relative percentage of motor units that are innervated by the motor nerve being tested. Amplitude of the SNAP response indicates the relative percentage of sensory nerve axons conducting the AP from the stimulation site to the recording electrodes. When recording over muscle, the amplitude is recording the size of the compound muscle action potential [measured in millivolts (mV)]. When recording over nerve (as in sensory nerve testing), the amplitude is recording the size of the nerve action potential [measured in micro-volts (uV)]. Using "supramaximal stimulation intensity" (see page 22) is very important to be sure all intact fibers are being depolarized and that the displayed AP is the most accurate reflection of the function of the nerve being tested.

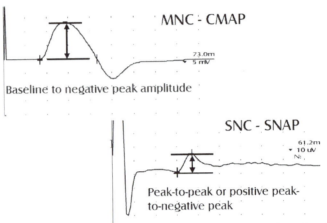

Figure 3-3: Amplitude of motor conduction testing (top) and SNAP (bottom). Photograph used with permission: Cadwell Laboratories, Inc.

Conduction Velocity (CV) refers to the speed of the AP along a segment of a nerve. Conduction velocity can be calculated along a peripheral nerve and estimated along tracts of the spinal cord. In order to calculate motor CV, you must stimulate at two separate locations along the nerve. For example, to test median nerve conduction in a patient with suspected carpal tunnel syndrome (CTS), the two sites of stimulation are the median nerve at the wrist and the elbow. The latency value from the wrist (to the Abductor Pollicis Brevis) and elbow are used, along with a measurement of the distance between the cathodes at the two sites of stimulation (wrist and elbow).

In Figure 3-4 (of someone with mild CTS), the top tracing was produced by stimulation at the elbow (elbow latency), and the bottom tracing is the wrist latency. Each box on the grid is 2ms horizontally, and 2.5mV vertically. At the left of each tracing is a small vertical line, which is the stimulus artifact. The initial deflections from baseline of the muscle depolarization are downward in this figure due to the active electrode being inserted into the positive down input jack on the preamplifier. The top tracing (elbow latency) travels 4 boxes (8ms) before deflecting downward, which is the beginning of the compound muscle action potential. The bottom (wrist latency) travels 2 boxes (4ms) before the slope changes and begins to form the same looking compound muscle action potential. Only the latency should change if you are recording from the same nerve & muscle.

The calculations below and to the right of the diagram show subtraction of the two latencies and the distance (25.9cm). The distance is converted to millimeters (259mm).
CV = distance/ longer latency - shorter latency
Calculations are elbow latency minus wrist latency
    8ms - 4ms = 4ms.

Conduction velocity (m/sec) = $\dfrac{\text{Distance (mm)}}{\text{T2 - T1 (ms)}}$

$$= \dfrac{259 \text{ mm}}{8\text{ms} - 4\text{ms}}$$

$$= \dfrac{259 \text{ mm}}{4\text{ms}} = 64.8\text{m/sec}$$

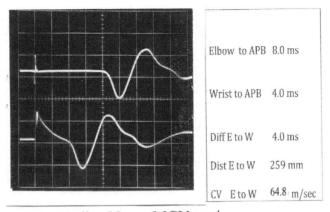

Figure 3-4: Median Nerve MCV testing

The overall duration of the CMAP reflects the conduction velocities of the different motor units. The most important component of this aspect of the test is the fastest conducting fibers. The wrist latency is used to assess the CV along the most distal segment of the nerve. You cannot measure between the site of stimulation and the active electrode over a muscle and calculate an accurate conduction velocity, due to the slowing of the AP along the unmyelinated terminal end fibers and the delay for the AP to cross the NMJ and produce a muscle contraction. There are normal values and other techniques for accurately interpreting the functioning of the most distal segment of a motor nerve.

Procedure for Testing & Clinical Decision Making
A thorough and complete initial evaluation is performed on any patient prior to initiating this testing. Testing is initiated if the initial evaluation reveals additional information is required to confirm or rule out a diagnosis. Based upon the results of the history and initial evaluation, a decision is made of which nerves should be tested. Results of each MCV or SNAP guide the examiner on what to examine in order to support a specific diagnostic hypothesis or rule it out. The standard testing protocols for each selected nerve

are followed unless alternate methods are necessary. For example, a patient with burns and scarring may need to be tested in alternate sites or with a needle into muscle. Skin preparation includes cleaning the area with alcohol wipes and lightly sanding the skin to reduce skin resistance prior to electrode placement.

Each individual or department that performs electroneuromyography testing has their specific set of normal values used for interpreting results of nerve conduction studies. Below is outlined one example of normal values used for interpretation.

Nerve	Segment	Latency (ms)	Significance	Segment	Velocity (m/sec)	Significance
Median	Wrist--> A.P.B.	<4.0 4.0 - 4.2 >4.2	Normal Borderline Prolonged	Elbow--> Wrist	> 50 47.5 - 50.0 <47.5	Normal Borderline Slow
Ulnar	Wrist--> A.D.Q.	<3.4 3.4 - 3.6 >3.6	Normal Borderline Prolonged	Elbow--> Wrist	Same as Above	Same as Above
Radial	Forearm-> Ext. Indicis	40.0 m/sec (velocity)	Normal	Spiral Groove -> Forearm	Same as above	Same as above

Table 3-1: UE Motor Conduction Studies - Interpretative Values

Interpretation of Values - Motor Conduction Studies
Significance of Abnormalities
- The distal latency (ex: wrist) is used to evaluate conduction from the most distal segment of the nerve to produce a CMAP in the muscle.
- If conduction velocity falls below 50m/second, all of the fastest conducting fibers are impaired. The overall duration of the CMAP will help reveal if temporal dispersion is present.
- This is most commonly due to demyelination or compression of the nerve axons in the area being tested.

- If a distal latency is prolonged, and the next proximal segment CV is normal, this is often due to distal compression.
- If the proximal segment CV is slow and the distal latency is prolonged, this reveals generalized demyelination.
- If the proximal segment is slow and the distal segment is normal, this is typically due to a compression lesion across the area where slowed CV was found. Testing for this will be discussed further in this chapter. Examples include pronator teres syndrome (compression as the median nerve passes through the two heads of the pronator teres) or tardy ulnar palsy (latent compression in the ulnar groove at the medial epicondyle).
- Axonal degeneration results in decreased amplitudes compared to decreased CV.
- Age affects nerve conduction velocity. Children below five years of age may have conduction velocity 50% lower than adults. Conduction velocity also decreases after middle age, but no more than 10m/second by age 60 or 80. Comparison to the "uninvolved" extremity is the best method of interpretation.

Median Nerve - Electrode Placement for Motor CV
Patient is positioned supine (Figure 3-5). The active electrode is placed over the belly of the Abductor Pollicis Brevis (APB). The reference electrode is placed distally over the tendon of the APB. The ground electrode is placed on the back of the palm. The first site of stimulation is at the wrist, using anatomical knowledge or landmarks such as between the tendons of the Flexor Carpi Radialis and the Palmaris Longus. Stimulator pulse duration is set at .05ms or .1ms and a frequency of once/second. Cathode is always the prong closest to the active electrode. As stimulus intensity is increased, the patient should be asked to report when they feel the stimulus in the distribution of the median nerve or the examiner should look for the beginnings of a

muscle twitch in the APB. At a low level of motor response, the examiner moves the stimulating electrodes medial or laterally to obtain the largest response. Then you know you are directly over the nerve. Turn up stimulator to supramaximal intensity as previously described. This confirms all nerve axons are being stimulated. Save the CMAP on the display, turn down the stimulator, and immediately mark the location of the cathode prong of the stimulator. You will later measure between the two cathode sites to determine the distance (length) of the nerve being tested. Repeat this procedure of stimulation at a second, more proximal site along the course of the median nerve (Figure 3-6). The second site of stimulation is anterior and just medial to the biceps tendon. The nerve is deeper at this location, but easily accessible. A third site of stimulation is in the upper arm as shown in Figure 3-6. This third site would be used when upper arm CV is also needed.

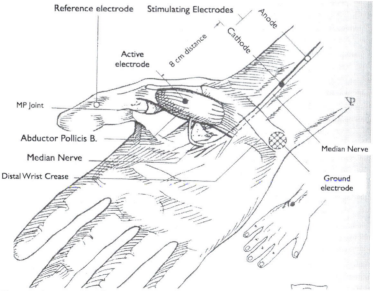

Figure 3-5: Median nerve recording sites and wrist stimulation site. (Diagram modified from NIOSH publication, 1990).

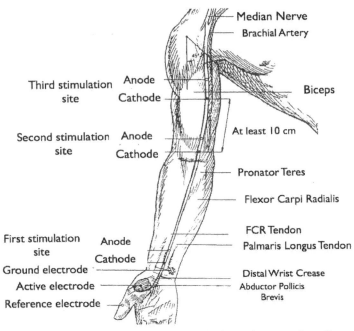

Figure 3-6: Median nerve stimulation sites at the elbow and upper arm. (Diagram modified from NIOSH publication, 1990).

Median Nerve Latencies & MVC's
Figure 3-7 shows tracings from the median nerve along the three sites described previously. The top sweep is stimulation at the wrist (O is the onset of the CMAP, P is measuring the peak). The middle sweep is produced with stimulation at the elbow, and the bottom sweep is with stimulation in the axilla. Confirmation that all three CMAP's are from the abductor pollicis brevis include identical waveforms except for the different latencies. The observed motor response in median nerve innervated muscles should be appropriate for each stimulation site. When stimulating at the wrist, only the thenar muscles should respond. When stimulating at the elbow (medial to the biceps tendon), all median nerve innervated muscles below the elbow should also respond, producing pronation, wrist and finger flexion.

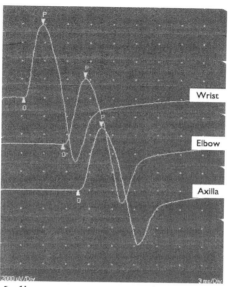

Figure 3-7: Median nerve compound muscle action potentials. Stimulation at the wrist, elbow and the axilla Photograph used with permission: Cadwell Laboratories, Inc.

Calculations for the median nerve testing above reveal:
Latency   Diff Lat   Distance   CV (d/t)
Wrist: 3.38ms   El - Wr=5.14   El-Wr 270mm   52m/sec
Elbow: 8.52ms   Ax - El =2.03   Ax-El 120mm   59m/sec
Axilla: 10.55ms

Median Nerve - Clinical Examples
CTS is one of the most common peripheral nerve compression syndromes. Clinical findings associated with CTS typically include sensory complaints limited to the median nerve distribution of the hand, normal sensation in the ulnar distribution and a positive Tinel's sign. The patient may complain of waking up at night with pins and needles in the hand and/or may complain of dropping objects from this hand. Additional clinical tests for CTS include a Phalen's

test and modified carpal compression test. Electrodiagnostic findings associated with CTS would include a prolonged wrist latency. Conduction velocity in the forearm (between elbow and wrist) should be normal, since the site of involvement is below that segment. Sensory testing will be described later in this chapter, and positive findings would include a prolonged latency of the SNAP and decreased amplitude. Sensory nerve changes occur prior to the onset of motor nerve changes.

If a person has pronator teres syndrome, then the CV through the forearm would typically be slowed if the fastest conducting motor fibers are affected, but the distal wrist latency would be normal (since CV is typically slowed only through the site of compression). If the compression is more severe and there is demyelination and axonal degeneration, then CV would be slow from the site of compression distally and the amplitude of the CMAP would be decreased compared to the amplitude attained from stimulation at the wrist. If there were only a partial conduction block at the site of compression, the result is a decreased amplitude of the CMAP, but with normal CV. CV testing for this patient should also include stimulation at the proximal third site, the axilla. This would allow for calculation of a CV from axilla to elbow, which should be normal in someone with compression in the forearm, as in pronator teres syndrome. By evaluating and showing normal CV above (and below) the site of compression helps to localize the site of compression.

Ulnar Nerve - Motor Conduction Studies
Patient is supine. The active electrode is placed over the belly of the Abductor Digiti Minimi (ADM) (Figure 3-8). The reference electrode is placed distally over its tendon and the ground electrode placed on the back of the palm, the same position as for median nerve testing. The first site of

stimulation is at the wrist, using anatomical knowledge or landmarks such as medial or lateral to the tendon of the flexor carpi ulnaris. This provides the wrist latency value. Stimulation parameters of pulse duration (.05 or .1), frequency (one pulse per second) and technique of confirming optimal stimulator position over the nerve is the same as described for the Median nerve.

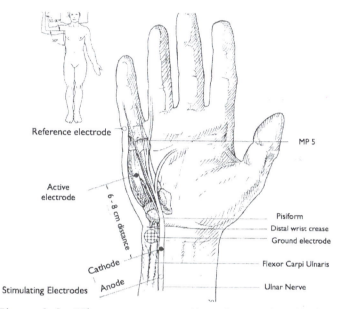

Figure 3-8: Ulnar nerve recording sites and wrist stimulation site. (Diagram modified from NIOSH publication, 1990).

The arm is abducted and the elbow flexed to 70-90 degrees (Figure 3-9). The ulnar nerve is on slack with the elbow extended. In order to produce an accurate measurement of the course of the nerve, it must be tested and measured with the elbow flexed at least 70 degrees. This position will produce an accurate representation of the nerve length when measured between the two stimulation sites of above the elbow and below the elbow. The tape measure is placed superficially along the course of the nerve following its course along the medial epicondyle as shown in Figure 3-9. To reduce calculation error, it is also very important that a minimum distance of 10 cm is maintained between any two points of nerve stimulation.

Conduction velocity in the forearm can be determined by stimulating the ulnar nerve at a second site just below the medial epicondyle. However, the most common site of ulnar nerve compression is in the ulnar groove at the medial epicondyle. Therefore, testing includes stimulating at four different sites along the course of the nerve (Figure 3-9). These sites are the wrist, below the medial epicondyle, above the medial epicondyle, and in the upper arm. This is referred to as an ulnar segmental MCV and allows calculation of CV along three nerve segments. The segments include:
- below elbow to wrist
- above elbow to below elbow (across the elbow)
- axilla to above elbow.

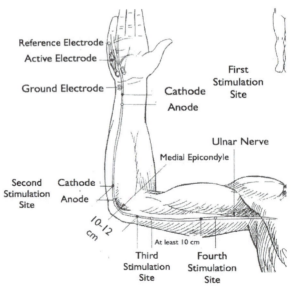

Figure 3-9: Ulnar nerve stimulation sites. (Diagram modified from NIOSH publication, 1990).

Figure 3-10 reveals what the compound muscle action potentials would look like when stimulating at each site, and how the conduction velocity is calculated for each segment. The active electrode is inserted into the negative-up input, resulting in an initial upward deflection of the CMAP.

The findings in this particular example reveal CV of 57m/sec above and below the elbow, but conduction velocity of 46 across the elbow. Interpretation of this data is two fold: conduction velocity across the elbow is more than 10m/sec slower than adjacent nerve segments, plus conduction velocity across the elbow is slower than 50m/sec. Either of these findings is indicative of localized compression in the area of the elbow. One of the many causes of ulnar nerve involvement in the elbow is due to positioning and weight bearing on the elbows. Other etiologies include prior fractures in the area of the medial epicondyle. After years of the ulnar nerve sliding up and down in the roughened post fracture ulnar groove, the nerve fibers get frayed like rope rubbing across a sharp surface. This pathology is referred to as a Tardy Ulnar Palsy. Patients with spinal cord injury or hemiplegia are also susceptible to ulnar nerve compression due to prolonged positioning in bed, in a wheelchair, or prolonged use of a lapboard without protecting the ulnar nerve at the elbow.

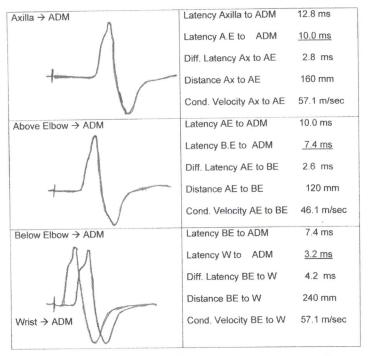

Figure 3-10: Ulnar segmental motor conduction studies. ADM = Abductor Digiti Minimi; Ax=Axilla; AE=Above Elbow; BE= Below Elbow; W=Wrist.

Ulnar nerve testing can also include assessment of the deep palmar branch of the ulnar nerve. This can be injured by direct trauma to the palm or compressed at the hook of the hamate. An example is cyclist's palsy. Stimulation is performed at the same wrist location, but with recording electrodes placed over the First Dorsal Interrossei (FDI) muscle. The latency to the FDI should not exceed the latency to the ADM by more than 2.0ms. A latency that exceeds this difference is indicative of nerve pathology in the deep palmar branch.

Radial Nerve - Motor Conduction Studies

Patient is supine. The arm is alongside the patient and pronated. The active electrode is placed over the belly of the Extensor Indicis (the most distally innervated muscle by the radial nerve). The reference electrode is placed distally over its tendon and the ground electrode is placed as shown in Figure 3-11.

The first site of stimulation is at the proximal forearm lateral to the extensor carpi ulnaris. The second site of stimulation is in the upper arm distal to the spiral groove, between the brachioradialis and the biceps. The third site of stimulation that can be used is in the axilla (Figure 3-12). This can allow calculation of CV along two sites, upper forearm and upper arm. Interpretation of the distal motor latency is an estimate based upon measuring the distance between the cathode of the first stimulation site and the active recording electrode. Since there is no specific landmark as there is with wrist stimulation (in median and ulnar nerve studies), the site of distal stimulation is very variable. Interpretation is via estimation of CV between the forearm stimulation site and active recording electrode, taking into account slowing that occurs in the distal fibers of the motor nerve, the NMJ, and the muscle action potential propagation. You will notice that the table for interpretation of Radial MCV's lists 40m/sec as borderline for normal, vs. 50 m/sec for all other UE nerve segments. EMG departments may have other interpretation methods for these findings.

Selection of stimulation sites is based upon the presentation of the patient and the desire to test multiple segments or just the distal segment of the nerve. If a patient had a history of a Colles fracture and numbness in the back of the hand, the problem may be due to an edematous arm in a cast or other etiologies that cause forearm compression and testing the first two sites is adequate. If a patient had a mid-humeral fracture or Saturday night palsy, then the concern is regarding the upper segment of the radial nerve, and more detailed testing is appropriate across the site of injury as well as distally. A mid-humeral fracture can result in direct radial nerve injury or delayed entrapment of the radial nerve in the callus formation of the healing humeral fracture.

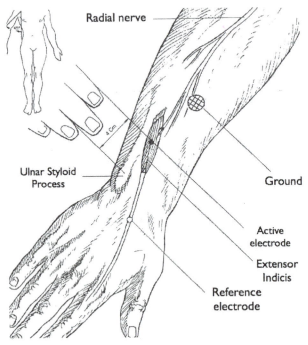

Figure 3-11: Radial nerve electrode placement. (Diagram modified from NIOSH publication, 1990).

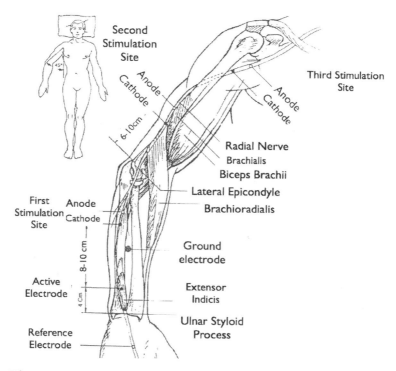

Figure 3-12: Radial nerve recording and stimulation sites at the elbow and upper arm. (Diagram modified from NIOSH publication, 1990).

Sensory Nerve Conduction Studies
Sensory Nerve Action Potentials (SNAPs). Refers to the measuring of a SNAP when stimulating a sensory nerve and recording the action potential from another site along the anatomical course of the nerve. Measurement is always of a pure nerve segment, so CV can be calculated between any two points of stimulation or between the stimulation site and the active recording electrode. However, CV is not the standard procedure due to the small size of the action potential and a greater possibility of error of measurement when low amplitude SNAP's occur.

Rationale for General Testing
- Most peripheral neuropathies affect sensory fibers before motor fibers.
- Evaluates the distal segment of a sensory nerve axon.
- Most sensory neuropathies start distally

SNAP's – Types of Electrodes & Recording Techniques
There are two types of electrodes that are most commonly used. A pair of stainless steel ring electrodes can be placed around one finger, distal to the PIP and DIP joints. A ground electrode is placed in the back of the hand as shown for motor conduction studies or in the diagram below. These ring electrodes can be used as recording electrodes or stimulating electrodes. If used as recording electrodes, the nerve being tested is stimulated at the wrist (as previously described for motor) and the nerve action is recorded over the finger innervated by that sensory nerve. This is Antidromic sensory nerve testing.

Ring electrodes can also be used to stimulate the sensory nerve fibers in one finger. The action potential will travel proximally (orthodromically) and can be recorded by placing a block electrode (shown in Chapter two) directly over the nerve at the wrist. The site of nerve stimulation for MCV's can be used to help determine the optimal location for this recording block electrode. The two metal prongs used for stimulation can be removed and the ends of the wires for the ring electrodes can be inserted into the stimulator. The recording electrodes are inserted into the amplifier with the electrode closest to the point of stimulation the active electrode and the second electrode the reference electrode.

Clinical Decision Making & Technique
- Where to place electrodes and why - UE testing typically includes Median and/or Ulnar nerves in routine screening. Orthodromic testing has advantages that

stimulation is occurring distally on one finger at a time, and therefore there is no activation of muscles and the possibility of volume conducted muscle responses contaminating the waveform seen.
- Skin preparation - proper technique for recording any biological potential includes lightly sanding the skin to reduce skin resistance and therefore improve accurate recording of the SNAP. The skin is also cleaned with an alcohol wipe.
- Recording electrodes should never be to close together that they might touch each other or that the gel applied to improve conduction will form an electrical bridge between the two recording electrodes.

A normal SNAP has a V shaped response. Some examiners use the initial deflection from baseline for measuring the latency, and others use the bottom of the V to measure the latency. Values listed below are using the initial deflection from baseline. The different conduction velocities of all sensory fibers in the nerve being tested produce the duration of the overall action potential. A U shaped response that has a longer duration, even if the initial latency is normal, is the first sign of mild nerve involvement. This is an example of temporal dispersion.

The amplitude of the SNAP is produced by a summation of the action potentials of all sensory fibers of the nerve. The amplitude is the first electrophysiological aspect of the test to typically reveal some nerve involvement. If 50% of the fibers are blocked by a neurapraxia (ex: CTS), then the amplitude of the SNAP will be reduced by 50%. However, the latency may still appear as normal since the other 50% of the fibers may be conducting normally, and reach the active electrode at the normal velocity.

When finding abnormalities in SNAP's, be sure that the abnormality is confirmed in more than one finger and that the other nerves of the UE are tested to determine if this is a mononeuropathy or polyneuropathy.

Nerve	Segment	Latency (ms)	Significance	Amplitude (uV)	Significance
Median	Wrist--> II, III	<3.6 ms 3.6 - 4.0 ms >4.0 ms	Normal Borderline Prolonged	> 15.0 10.0 - 15.0 <10.0	Normal Borderline Low
Ulnar	Wrist--> V	<3.4 ms 3.4 - 4.0 ms >4.0 ms	Normal Borderline Prolonged	Same as Above	Same as Above
Radial	Forearm-> wrist	Cond. Velocity >50.0 m/sec 47.5 - 50.0 m/sec <47.5 m/sec	Normal Borderline Prolonged	Same as above	Same as above

Table 3-2: UE SNAPs – Interpretative values – U. E.

SNAP's – Significance of Abnormalities
- Low Amplitude SNAP – partial axonal degeneration and/or partial compression.
- Prolonged Latency SNAP – demyelination or more moderate compression.
- Absent response – more severe compression or axonal degeneration.

Median Nerve SNAP - Electrode Placement & Technique
Examples are shown of both antidromic (Figure 3-13) and orthodromic testing (Figure 3-14). In antidromic, the stimulator is held at the wrist, the ground is just distal to the stimulator and the active and reference electrodes are on the second digit. In orthodromic testing, the setup may look the same, but stimulating and recording electrodes are reversed.

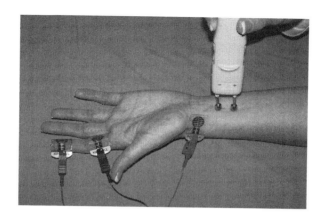

Figure 3-13: Antidromic median nerve SNAP setup. Photograph used with permission: Cadwell Laboratories, Inc.

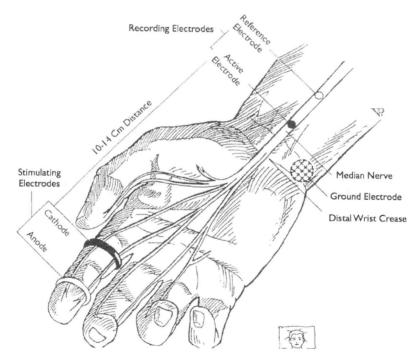

Figure 3-14: Orthodromic median nerve SNAP setup (Diagram modified from NIOSH publication, 1990).

Figure 3-15 is from antidromic SNAP's in a patient with CTS. The initial deflection is downward due to the active electrode being inserted into the positive-down input jack of the preamplifier. The SNAP's are low amplitude (8-10uV) and borderline prolonged duration (3.6 - 4.0msec). Amplifier settings are 10uV/vertical division and 2ms per horizontal division. The baselines are thick due to the high level of amplification to assist in visualizing the beginning of the response in order to measure the latency value. The latency is determined by analyzing each sweep for a change in the slope after the stimulus artifact to the beginning of the downward deflection. You should note that if the latency value used was to the peak of the downward deflection, the latency would be more accurate for comparison to normal values (when measuring latency to the peak of the SNAP versus the initial take off). You will be able to compare these to the normal SNAP's in the ulnar nerve (on p. 50) and readily observe the differences.

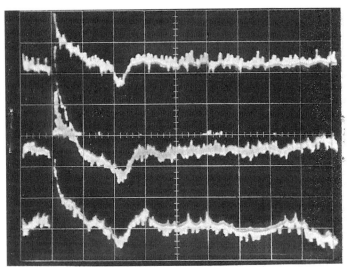

Figure 3-15: Antidromic median nerve SNAP's - CTS

Ulnar Nerve SNAP - Electrode Placement & Technique
Figure 3-16 shows orthodromic testing. The ring electrodes are serving as the stimulating electrodes, and a block recording electrode would be placed over the ulnar nerve at the wrist, using the landmarks from the ulnar motor latency stimulation site. The block electrode can also be first attached to the stimulator, and using low levels of stimulation, determine the optimal location for depolarizing the nerve (via the patient's reported sensations in the hand or using the lowest intensity to produce a motor response. Then insert the block electrode wires into the amplifier.

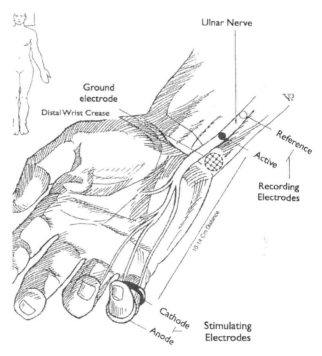

Figure 3-16: Orthodromic Ulnar Nerve SNAP Setup (Diagram modified from NIOSH publication, 1990).

Figure 3-17 displays shows two tracings from antidromic ulnar SNAP's of the same patient. Settings are 20uV/vertical division and 2/ms horizontal division. The break in the sweep (at 2ms) is the stimulus artifact, the V is the SNAP, and the continuous waveform afterward is a volume conducted motor response. The latency (2.0-2.1msec) and amplitude (31uV) are both normal.

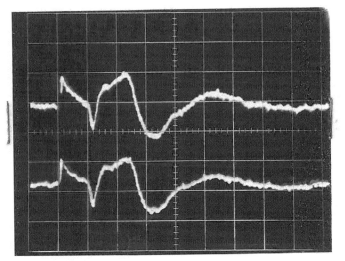

Figure 3-17: Antidromic ulnar SNAP's. Same patient in Fig 3-16.

Radial Nerve SNAP - Electrode Placement & Technique
Active and reference electrodes are placed directly over the Superficial Branch of the Radial Nerve, located via landmarks and palpation over an extended Extensor Pollicis Longus tendon (Figures 3-18 & 3-19). A different method is to place recording ring electrodes over the posterior aspect of the thumb. The stimulation site is located using landmarks and palpation as shown. Dividing the latency value by the distance between the active electrode and the stimulating cathode electrode makes calculation of CV easy.

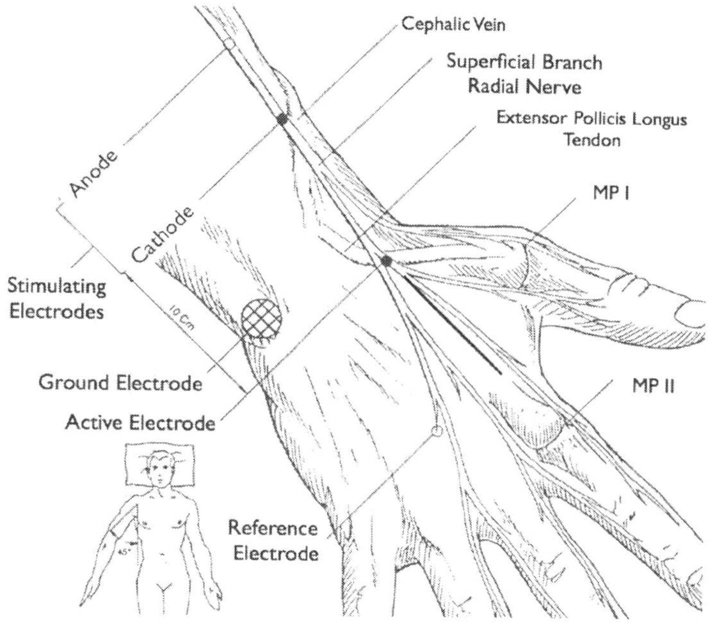

Figure 3-18: Antidromic superficial radial SNAP. (Diagram modified from NIOSH publication, 1990).

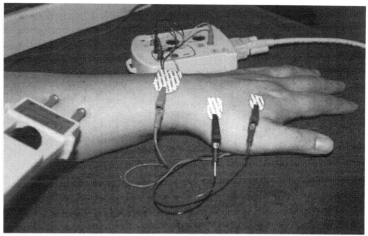

Figure 3-19: Antidromic superficial radial SNAP Photograph used with permission: Cadwell Laboratories, Inc.

Figures 3-20 & 3-21 are examples of Radial nerve SNAP's. In both figures, there are three tracings, with the upward deflection being the SNAP. Vertical boxes are 20uV each and horizontal boxes are 1ms. Figure 3-20, the left radial antidromic SNAP reveals an onset latency of 1.5ms and an amplitude of 40uV (top and middle tracing) - 50uV (bottom tracing).

In Figure 3-21, the left radial orthodromic SNAP reveals an onset latency of 1.5ms and amplitudes in the range of 35uV.

The values in these figures are all WNL's in both latency and amplitude. Multiple tracings reveal good consistency in latency values, and some variability in the amplitude. The difference in results reflects differences between antidromic testing (stimulating in distal forearm/wrist) and orthodromic (stimulating at anatomical stuffbox).

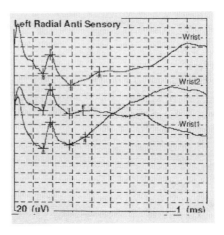

Figure 3-20: Antidromic superficial branch of radial N. Photograph used with permission: Cadwell Laboratories, Inc.

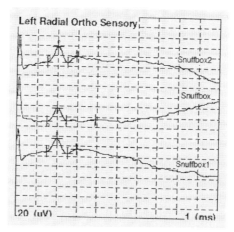

Figure 3-21: Orthodromic superficial branch of radial N. Photograph used with permission: Cadwell Laboratories, Inc.

CHAPTER FOUR

Lower Extremity Motor Nerve Conduction Studies & Sensory Nerve Action Potential's

Upon completion of this chapter, the reader will:

- Be able to explain the rationale for performing motor nerve and sensory nerve conduction testing of peripheral nerves of the lower extremity (LE).
- Be able explain the selection of the most appropriate tests of the LE based upon the potential diagnosis of the patient.
- Be able to describe and explain the technique for performing motor and sensory nerve conduction studies on the fibular, tibial, and sural nerves.
- Be able to interpret the results of these tests based upon normal values to assist in the eventual diagnosis of the patient.
- determine the location of a peripheral nerve lesion, estimate the extent of this lesion, and determine the need for additional nerve conduction studies and EMG.

Evaluation of the lower extremity nerves is based upon the same rationale, equipment, electrodes, technique, and interpretation as previously described for the upper extremities. Normal values are different and are outlined below.

A patient developing a polyneuropathy usually presents with lower extremity involvement prior to UE involvement. Therefore, testing the LE's first is appropriate and more helpful to guide the remainder of the evaluation.

Motor Nerve Conduction Studies

Conduction velocity (CV) reveals velocity of the fastest conducting fibers and amplitude reveals the relative number of muscle fibers or motor units that are innervated. Compared to the UE, the LE distal latencies are longer, and conduction velocity is normally slower than in the UE. The literature is unclear on the reason for slower CV in the LE's compared to the UE's. Temperature of the LE is lower, but not adequate to explain the 10m/sec difference. Proximal segments in the LE conduct faster than distal segments, and this may also due to decreases in internodal distances and decreased diameter of distal nerve axons. The table below displays a set of normal values for motor latencies and conduction velocity.

Nerve	Segment	Latency (ms)	Significance	Amplitude (uV)	Significance
Superficial Fibular	Leg --> Foot	Cond. Velocity > 40.0 m/sec 37.5 - 40.0 m/sec <37.5 m/sec	Normal Borderline Prolonged	> 10.0 8.0 - 10.0 < 8.0	Normal Borderline Low
Sural	Calf --> Ankle	Cond. Velocity > 40.0 m/sec 37.5 - 40.0 m/sec <37.5 m/sec	Normal Borderline Prolonged	Same as Above	Same as Above

Table 4-1: LE motor conduction studies - Interpretative values.

Significance of Abnormalities

If conduction velocity falls below 40m/second, the fastest conducting motor fibers are impaired, as occurs in demyelination. Compression of all of the fastest conducting fibers will also result in a decreased CV. Neuropathic or myopathic disease can affect the amplitude of the CMAP. Axonal degeneration or loss of muscle fibers will result in a proportional decrease in amplitude. Prolonged distal latencies, as in the UE, are often associated with distal compression.

Testing Deep Fibular Nerve

The active electrode is placed over the belly of the Extensor Digitorum Brevis (EDB), which is one of two intrinsic muscles of the foot innervated by this nerve. Whenever possible, the most distally innervated muscle should be selected as the recording site. This allows testing of the most distal segment of the nerve. The reference electrode is placed distally beyond the belly of the muscle. The ground electrode can be placed as shown or another location between the stimulation site and active electrode. The first site of stimulation is deep in the anterior ankle, just lateral to the tendons of the Tibialis Anterior and the Extensor Hallucis Longus. The result will yield a CMAP of the EDB and measurement of the ankle latency. The following figures display the set-up of electrodes and stimulation sites.

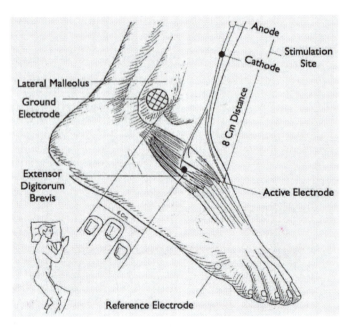

Figure 4-1: Deep Fibular Nerve – Electrode placement and ankle latency. (Diagram modified from NIOSH publication, 1990).

The second site of stimulation (see Figure 4-2) is just below the head of the fibula, which provides a second latency value, used in calculating the CV from below the knee to the ankle. If compression at the head of the fibula is being considered, then stimulation at a third site, deep in the lateral border of the popliteal fossa, will allow calculation of a CV of the nerve segment above the head of the fibula to below the head of the fibula. This site of compression is more common than some clinicians realize, especially in patients who have sustained a severe stroke, positioning problems with the leg externally rotated and resultant pressure on the lateral aspect of the lower leg. Direct trauma can also result in nerve damage. A normal ankle latency, normal CV in the lower leg, and slow CV across the fibula head would confirm localized compression at the fibula head.

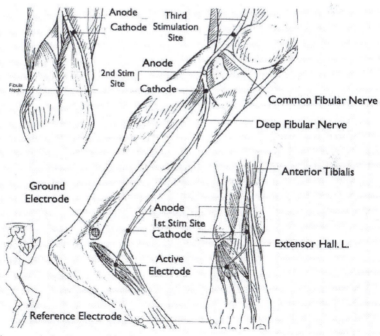

Figure 4-2: Deep fibular nerve - MCV. (Diagram modified from NIOSH publication, 1990).

Fibular Nerve MVC's

The example shown in Figure 4-3 is a typical printout from computer-based equipment. The settings are included, which is important for data collection. These settings include the amplification, filter settings, stimulator pulse width, sweep speed, and rate of stimulation. The equipment presets the settings when a specific nerve test is selected from a menu. Two tracings are shown. The top is was produced with stimulation at the ankle (ankle latency is 3.53ms), and the bottom is with stimulation at the knee (knee latency is 9.77ms). The difference in knee to ankle latency is 6.24ms. The two vertical lines and arrows are the computer-assisted measurements of these two latencies. By entering the distance between the two cathode stimulating electrodes (36 cm or 360mm), the conduction velocity is automatically calculated, revealing a NCV of 57.69m/sec. These results are within normal limits.

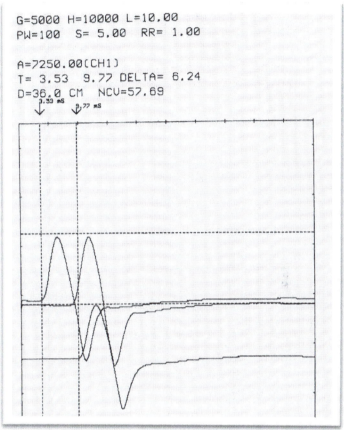

Figure 4-3: Fibular Nerve - Examples of NCV.

Testing the Posterior Tibial Nerve

The Abductor Hallucis (AH) muscle is used as the primary recording site. Refer to Figure 4-4 for visual landmarks. The AH is located along the medial longitudinal arch and easily accessible with surface electrodes. The active electrode is placed over the belly of the muscle, and the reference electrode is placed distally and laterally, to avoid placement over callus skin on the plantar surface of the foot. The ground electrode can often remain in the same location as in testing the Fibular nerve. The distal stimulation site is along the medial aspect of the lower leg, between the tendon of the gastrocnemius and the medial malleolus. Stimulation at this site and recording the CMAP over the AH provides determination of the ankle latency for the Tibial nerve. Prolonged distal tibial nerve latencies are highly indicative of Tarsal Tunnel Syndrome.

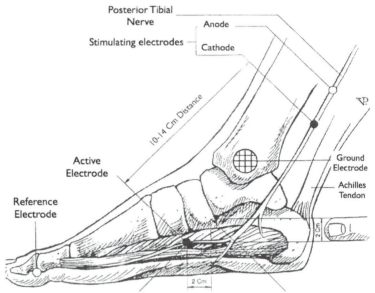

Figure 4-4: Posterior tibial nerve - Ankle setup. (Diagram modified from NIOSH publication, 1990).

Performing a Posterior Tibial Nerve MCV
The second site of stimulation is deep and in the midline of the popliteal fossa, between the medial and lateral gastrocnemius tendons. In many individuals, stimulation of the nerve requires a longer pulse duration due to the increased depth of the tibial nerve at this site. Supramaximal stimulation will produce a strong plantarflexion contraction and CMAP of the AH to confirm the nerve is being activated optimally.

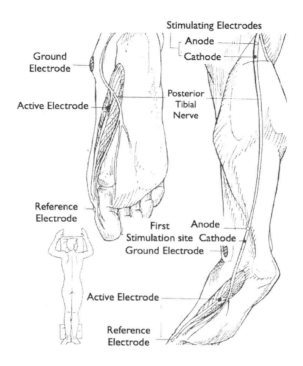

Figure 4-5: Posterior tibial nerve - Stimulation and recording sites. (Diagram modified from NIOSH publication, 1990).

Motor Conduction Studies – Tibial Nerve
Below are two examples of the results of Tibial nerve testing. Both are WNL. In each screen, the shape of the CMAP is the same except for the difference in latency. This consistency is very important to confirm that the tibial nerve is being stimulated at both points and conducting to the AH and therefore producing the identical CMAP. The amplitudes in figure 4-6 vary due to the stimulation being below or at supramaximal intensity (performed by students on each other for initial testing experience).

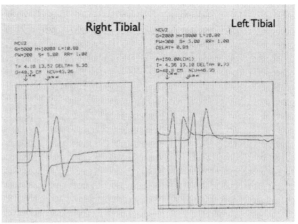

Figure 4-6: Posterior Tibial Nerve - NCV Studies

The display labeled Right Tibial nerve reveals an ankle latency of 4.16ms, a knee latency of 13.52ms and the difference (Delta) of 9.36ms. The distance between the two points of stimulation (knee to ankle) was 40.5 cm. Calculation of a CV was 43.26 m/sec. All these values are WNL.

The display labeled Left Tibial nerve reveals an ankle latency of 4.36ms, a knee latency of 13.10ms and the difference (Delta) of 8.73ms. The distance between the two stimulation points (knee to ankle) was 40.5 cm. Calculation of a CV was 46.35 m/sec. All values are WNL.

Sensory Nerve Conduction Studies
Rationale for testing
- This is the same decision making as in performing a clinical evaluation.
- Most systemic neuropathies begin in the Lower Extremities.
- Most peripheral neuropathies initially affect sensory fibers before motor fibers.

- Most sensory neuropathies start distally; therefore testing the most distal segment increases the sensitivity of the evaluation.

Clinical Decision Making

Determining where to begin the electrodiagnostic testing is based upon the results of the initial evaluation. SNAP testing of the LE's may be the first component of the examination. As a review, sensory nerve fibers tend to be affected in most peripheral polyneuropathies prior to motor fibers being affected, and the lower extremities are most commonly affected first due to their greater length and exposure to systemic pathological conditions.

Nerve	Segment	Latency (ms)	Significance	Amplitude (uV)	Significance
Superficial Fibular	Leg --> Foot	Cond. Velocity > 40.0 m/sec 37.5 - 40.0 m/sec <37.5 m/sec	Normal Borderline Prolonged	> 10.0 8.0 - 10.0 < 8.0	Normal Borderline Low
Sural	Calf --> Ankle	Cond. Velocity > 40.0 m/sec 37.5 - 40.0 m/sec <37.5 m/sec	Normal Borderline Prolonged	Same as Above	Same as Above

Table 4-2: LE SNAP - Interpretative Values

SNAP's – Significance of Abnormalities

Results of testing appear very similar to UE SNAP's. The distal segment is always the most revealing in someone with suspected peripheral neuropathy.
- Low amplitude SNAP – axonal loss, partial compression and/or demyelination (with associated conduction block).
- Prolonged latency SNAP – moderate compression, such as Tarsal Tunnel Syndrome.
- Absent response – more severe.

Superficial Fibular Nerve - Electrode Placement

In the lower extremities, testing is always done antidromically. Recording electrodes are placed over the sensory nerve fibers using anatomical landmarks and palpation. Figure 4-7 reveals landmarks and electrode placement.

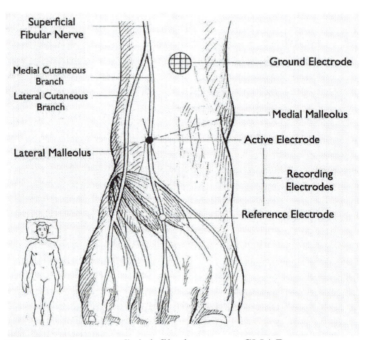

Figure 4-7: Superficial fibular nerve SNAP setup. (Diagram modified from NIOSH publication, 1990).

Figure 4-8 displays lower leg landmarks including the site of stimulation along the anterior lateral aspect of the lower leg, anterior to the fibularis longus tendon. This is strictly a sensory branch, so there is no motor response to help confirm being over the nerve and observing a CMAP.

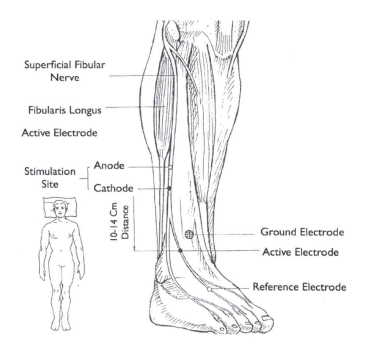

Figure 4-8: Superficial fibular nerve - Recording & stimulation site. (Diagram modified from NIOSH publication, 1990).

Sural Nerve - Electrode placement and Stimulation Sites
The sural nerve is a pure sensory nerve with its distribution in the lower foot and ankle. Electrode placement and stimulation sites are based upon anatomical landmarks as shown below in Figure 4-9. The active electrode is placed inferior to the lateral malleolus and the reference electrode is distally as shown. The stimulation site is at least 14 cm proximal to the active electrode, just distal and lateral to the gastrocnemius tendon. This (along with other tests) is an important nerve to evaluate in the early diagnosis of suspected diabetic neuropathy.

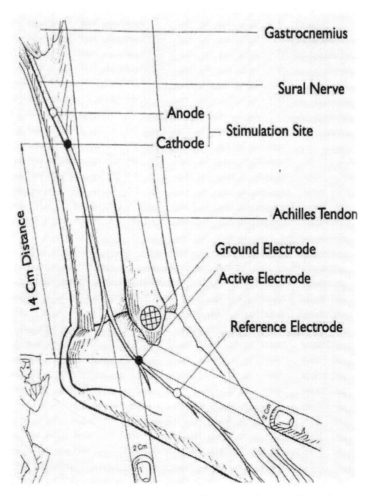

Figure 4-9: Sural Nerve - Recording & stimulation site. (Diagram modified from NIOSH publication, 1990).

CHAPTER FIVE

Advanced Techniques of Nerve Studies - Late Responses

Upon completion of this chapter, the reader will be able to describe the indications for, correct procedure, and interpretation of:
- Somatosensory Evoked Potentials
- Brainstem Auditory Evoked Potentials
- Visual Evoked Potentials
- H - Reflex
- F - Wave
- Repetitive Nerve Stimulation

There are various conditions in which these advanced techniques are beneficial in the diagnostic process. Standard nerve conduction studies assess for compression, demyelination and/or axonal degeneration of peripheral nerves, but are unable to assess the more proximal segments of the peripheral nervous system. Some of the tests described in this chapter provide an objective assessment of the conductivity and intactness of the sensory tracts of the spinal cord, cranial nerves and certain CNS pathways. Other tests evaluate NMJ function and proximal segments of peripheral nervous system. Coupled with standard nerve conduction studies, the entire peripheral nervous system and some components of the CNS can be assessed.

Somatosensory Evoked Potentials (SSEP's)
This test allows the examiner to evaluate conduction along proximal segments of the peripheral nervous system and the posterior columns of the spinal cord (SC), including pathways to the Primary Sensory Cortex in the Parietal lobe. For example, in a trauma center, the physicians need to evaluate a patient with a possible spinal cord injury. The patient is unconscious and/or heavily medicated and/or they

need an objective measure of nerve conduction within the spinal cord. Performing SSEP's can assess the conduction of action potentials along the sensory tracts of the SC to determine if they are compromised, blocked, or hopefully, intact. To test conduction through the Lumbar or Thoracic SC, stimulation is performed in a LE peripheral nerve. To test the Cervical SC, stimulation is performed on the median or ulnar nerve at the wrist. A block stimulating electrode is placed over the mixed nerve and recording (EEG needles) electrodes are placed subcutaneously over the sensory cortex (on the opposite hemisphere) that corresponds to the peripheral area being stimulated. The primary sensory cortex for the hand is located laterally in the sensory homunculus and the sensory cortex for the foot is medially oriented. A specialized computer averager is used with the EMG machine to allow recording of these very small AP's through the skull (remember volume conduction?). The AP is consistently of the same latency (unless absent), while random electrical noise will average out to zero. The computer displays the averaged SSEP signal and the examiner can determine the amplitude and latency of the SSEP and compare this to normal values. All parameters of the SSEP are evaluated, including the amplitudes, latencies and temporal dispersion. Abnormalities or absent responses have the same diagnostic implications as they do in testing the extremities. One example of normal values for the initial latency for SSEP's is 14-18 ms latency for the upper extremities and 23-31 ms latency value for the lower extremities. Please note that different testing centers use slightly different normal values. This includes whether the latency is measured to the beginning of the response or the initial peak of the response.

As shown in Figure 5-1, the top waveform is showing an upper extremity SSEP of 19ms latency. N19 refers to the waveform having a negative peak and the 19 refer to the latency measurement to the peak in milliseconds. Since the median nerve has mixed size fibers, there are multiple phases (positive and negative) corresponding to the CV of these different sensory fibers. P22 refers to the positive peak, which occurred at a latency of 22ms.

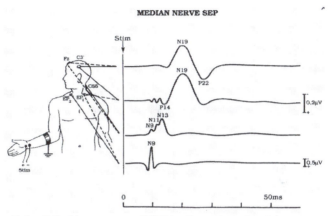

Figure 5-1: Median nerve SSEP. Reprinted with permission: Electrodiagnosis and Rehabilitation Associates of Tacoma, P.S., Tacoma, WA.

SSEP's can also be used to evaluate conduction through the brachial plexus or other proximal segments. Recording electrodes can also be placed over Erb's point (EP in the above diagram) and/or over C5 to measure latencies to these anatomical points. Abnormal values (latency and/or amplitude) at these points can assist in the diagnosis of brachial plexus compression, thoracic outlet syndrome, root compression or generalized proximal demyelination.

Other examples of the clinical/diagnostic implications for SSEP's include using this technique to monitor the SC during spinal surgery. A patient having scoliosis correction surgery is having their SC straightened during the surgery, and then stabilization devices inserted. Straightening the cord involves some degree of traction, and traction can result in decreased blood flow to the SC if performed to aggressively. Performing pre-operative SSEP's gives a baseline and then performing SSEP's during surgery can allow for close monitoring of the effect of the surgery on SC integrity. With optimal realignment, the amplitude of the SSEP may actually increase, but with overly aggressive correction or injury to the tracts, the SSEP parameters would decline immediately and allow the surgeon to prevent serious injury by reducing the amount of correction. SC monitoring like this is appropriate for any invasive spinal cord surgery.

Brainstem Auditory Evoked Potentials (BAER's)
The pathways of the auditory system can be evaluated for conductivity in a similar manner to SSEP's. Audiologists are also specifically trained in the use of this diagnostic procedure. Placing headphones on a client and using clicks to produce auditory stimulation of the cochlea, results in the production of action potentials that travel along the auditory pathways to the primary auditory cortex. Testing is performed unilaterally. Computer averaging is used as described in performing SSEP's, and results in a measurable waveform revealing amplitude and latency while recording over the ipsilateral temporal lobe. Acoustic neuroma is one example of a lesion that can result in cochlear nerve damage. However, unilateral partial damage beyond the brainstem will not cause deafness in one ear, since the afferent signals project bilaterally from the brainstem.

Visually Evoked Potentials (VEP's)
Stimulation with special goggles that produce a strobe-like visual stimulus is used to evaluate the pathways of the visual system. Recording electrodes are placed over the primary occipital cortex and will pick up the AP from each visual stimuli using computer averaging as described previously. VEP's can be performed unilaterally or bilaterally. All parameters of the VEP are evaluated for abnormal values

that reflect possible demyelination, compression or other pathological changes to the visual pathways. Abnormalities of the VEP will only localize the site of the lesion to the visual pathways between the optic nerve and the occipital lobe.

H- Reflex
The H-reflex is the electrical equivalent of the deep tendon reflex (DTR). When using DTR's to evaluate a patient, you are activating the spindle apparatus, evaluating the conductivity of the Ia afferent fibers, the responsiveness of the anterior horn cells and the conduction of the motor fibers innervating the muscle tested. Performing a H-reflex involves stimulating a motor nerve but rather than examine the CMAP directly (orthodromically), you are evaluating conduction along the pathways of the DTR. The test allows objective measure of all parameters of this AP.

The technique involves, for example:
- Recording electrodes are placed over the medial and lateral gastrocnemius.
- Stimulating the tibial nerve at the popliteal fossa.
- Ignore the immediate orthodromic motor response. The H reflex is the second waveform with a longer latency. This is produced by the action potential, which travels orthodromically in the sensory fibers to the SC and activates the anterior horn cell to discharge and produce a second depolarization, which travels orthodromically in motor fibers to the gastrocnemius muscle. The CMAP of the gastrocnemius is the H-reflex.
- This evaluates conduction along the entire pathway – orthodromic sensory and motor fibers associated with that reflex.
- Low intensity stimulation is used.

Figure 5-2 shows testing the H reflex of the tibial nerve. The active electrode is placed on one belly of the gastrocnemius muscle, the reference electrode (Ref) is placed distally off the muscle, and a ground electrode (Gr) is placed between the active electrode and the stimulation site. The tibial nerve is stimulated with the cathode proximally on the nerve. The display includes two waveforms. The first is the CMAP, produced by the AP travelling from the stimulator directly to the muscle. This waveform is not measured. The second waveform (H-reflex) becomes visible as the orthodromic sensory AP is of an intensity above threshold to activate the AHC's of the gastrocnemius. The amplitude, latency and overall waveform configuration should be almost equivalent to the other side in a healthy individual. Average latency for the gastrocnemius H-reflex is 29ms in an adult and there should be less than a 2ms difference between the contralateral muscles. Delay in the latency tends to reflect demyelination or compression along the pathway (ex: root compression) and decreased amplitude is associated with axonal loss or a partial conduction block. This test can be used to help diagnose proximal disease processes in peripheral nerves or nerve root compression that cannot be tested directly with standard peripheral nerve testing procedures.

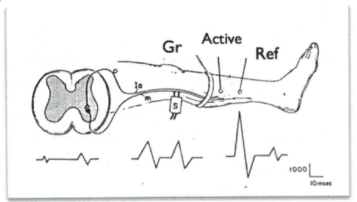

Figure 5-2: H - Reflex

F- Wave Testing

F-Waves are performed with the identical set-up as in performing the H-reflex. Almost any distal muscle in either extremity can have this reflex testing performed. The difference in technique is the intensity of the stimulation is supramaximal, compared to low levels of stimulation used for the H-reflex. During this procedure of testing for the F-wave, as stimulation is increased above threshold for the nerve fibers, the CMAP appears, followed by the H-Reflex. As the intensity of stimulation continues to be increased, the H-Reflex will be blocked and disappear. With increased intensity of stimulation, a second waveform will again appear. This waveform is produced by antidromic conduction along the motor fibers, followed by backfiring of the AHC, which produces an orthodromic motor outflow down the nerve to the muscle. This second twitch in the muscle is the F-wave and can be seen in Figure 5-3 above the arrow. F-wave testing is less sensitive in revealing mild compression as in radiculopathies or entrapment syndromes, but is more sensitive in revealing proximal involvement in Guillian Barre Syndrome, diabetic and other neuropathies with proximal involvement, or spinal cord/AHC involvement. Normal values vary depending upon the stimulation and record site, and therefore interpretation should be based upon the values provided by the examiner.

In summary, F-Wave testing:
- Tests conduction antidromically and orthodromically of the motor axons.
- Evaluates the excitability of the AHC.
- F wave will increase in amplitude with spasticity.
- F wave will decrease in amplitude or be absent in spinal shock or motor neuron disease (ex: polio, ALS, spinal muscular atrophy).

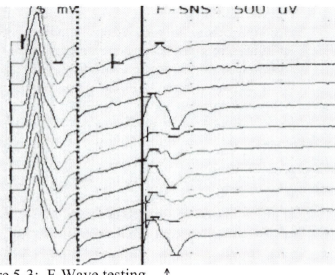

Figure 5-3: F-Wave testing ↑

Repetitive Nerve Stimulation (RNS) - Myasthenia Gravis
Evaluation of a patient with possible Myasthenia Gravis (MG) requires a very specific assessment of the neuromuscular junction. Manifestations of MG include; abnormal weakness after repetitive or sustained muscular effort, recovery after rest, weakness in extraocular, cervical and/or shoulder girdle muscles and ptosis is a very common early manifestation.

Testing procedure: Limb temperature in evaluating for MG is very important and must be maintained at normal values prior to testing. Recording electrodes are either a small EEG needle or disposable self-adhesive electrodes. The active electrode must be in (or over) the belly of the muscle, and the second reference electrode placed over the tendon. A ground electrode is placed between the point of stimulation and recording. Testing should include proximal and distal sites, such as an intrinsic hand muscle (ADM), proximal muscle (Deltoid) and one facial muscle (Orbicularis Oculi). Stimulating electrodes are secured over the nerve as in typical distal motor latencies or using a needle subcutaneously. The bar electrodes (Fig. 2-1) are excellent for stimulating the nerve because it can be firmly secured to the extremity with an elastic strap or elastic Dermaclear® tape. If the hand is being tested, the wrist/hand should be stabilized on a padded firm surface.

- Repetitive nerve stimulation (RNS) is performed at various frequencies (2, 3, 5, 50 Hz). Low frequencies of stimulation require a total of only six stimuli. High frequency requires one second of stimuli.
- Various methods of recording are recommended, either very slow sweep speeds (200msec/division) or 2msec/division. The slower allows examination of the overall amplitude change, while the faster speed allows visual examination of each CMAP for measurement and comparison of the CMAP amplitude of each waveform.

Intensity of stimulation (supramaximal) is the same as in NCV testing, to insure that all motor units are being activated. RNS begins at 2 pulses per second (pps). Each action potential displayed (in Figure 5-4) is with a sweep speed of five milliseconds per division and shows a normal configuration with no change in the peak-to-peak amplitude.

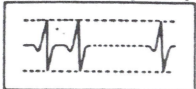

Figure 5-4: Repetitive Stimulation at 2 pps.

Figure 5-5 shows the results of RNS at 50 pulses per second. In a healthy person, there may be a very mild decrease in peak-to-peak amplitude or no decrease.

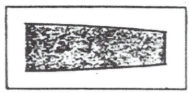

Figure 5-5: Repetitive Stimulation at 50 pps. (Normal)

Figure 5-6 reveals the results of RNS at 50 pulses per second in a patient with Myasthenia Gravis. There is an immediate and continuous decline in the amplitude of the compound muscle action potentials.

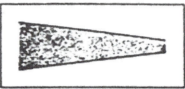

Figure 5-6: Repetitive Stimulation at 50 pps. (MG)

Results: Normal decreases in amplitude of the CMAP vary in the literature with most sources reporting decreases up to 12%. This varies between males and females and proximal versus distal muscles, with proximal muscles having higher diagnostic sensitivity. Each diagnostic laboratory has their own specific guidelines for interpretation of results.

If the results reveal a decrease in amplitude of greater than 10% at more than one site, this implies a high probability of a diagnosis of MG. At low rates of stimulation, a decrement in amplitude is obvious when comparing the amplitude of the first CMAP to the following five CMAP's. Decreases in amplitude with both low and high rates of stimulation help confirm the diagnosis of MG. If a physician is performing this examination, an excellent confirming test is the injection of a medication that is an anticholinergic drug after the initial series of RNS reveals findings consistent with MG. A repeat RNS which is normal after administration of this drug confirms the diagnosis.

Summary: SSEP's, H-reflex and F wave testing allow assessment of previously described proximal segments of the peripheral nervous system and the sensory pathways of the spinal cord. Additional examples of where this testing might be appropriate to rule in or rule out a diagnosis include the following, which would be followed by diagnostic EMG:

- Piriformis Syndrome - standard nerve conduction studies do not test across this site of compression of the sciatic nerve. SSEP's, H-reflex, F-wave testing can all be used to assess the sciatic nerve in this region. Testing the peripheral nerve segments and finding normal results helps to place the focus of involvement proximally when these advanced tests reveal abnormal findings. A more focused diagnosis can be made when combined with clinical assessment and EMG, which will be presented in chapter six.

- Thoracic Outlet Syndrome (TOS) - consists of two different classifications, vascular and neurological etiology. Standard nerve conduction studies do not test across the thoracic outlet. Median and ulnar motor and sensory conduction studies, ulnar segmental NCV's, SSEP and F wave testing, may help to determine the presence of TOS. When coupled with clinical provocative tests and imaging, a clearer diagnosis of TOS can be determined. Classically, results should rule out involvement below the thoracic outlet, while revealing findings suggestive of proximal involvement. However, the double crush theory of McComas revealed that patients with proximal nerve compression could cause more distal sites along the nerve to be more susceptible to compression. Clinically, this may present as a patient presenting with CTS concurrent with TOS, or Cervical radiculopathy with TOS, but the clinical assuming it was the more common disorder, and not

TOS. Differential diagnosis of TOS is complex and beyond the scope of this section. Whether the diagnosis is clear or not, unless a structural etiology (such as a cervical rib) is confirmed at the etiology, surgical intervention should not be considered as a first choice. Physical therapy has been shown to be an effective first intervention to correct mal-alignment that may be compressing neurovascular structures in the thoracic outlet.

CHAPTER SIX

Diagnostic Electromyography

Upon completion of this chapter, the reader will be able to:
- describe the indications for referring a patient for and/or performing diagnostic EMG.
- correctly interpret any component of a diagnostic EMG examination.
- explain the significance of normal and abnormal waveforms seen in a diagnostic EMG examination.
- describe how a diagnostic EMG can assist in determining the prognosis for a patient with nerve pathology.

Diagnostic electromyography (EMG) is the last and the most important component of an electroneuromyography examination. Diagnostic EMG is a method of examining the electrical waveform of each motor unit, similar to how an ECG displays and allows examination of cardiac muscle. Prior testing procedures help to determine the conductivity of the peripheral (and central) nervous system, and reveal if localized compression, demyelination and/or axonal degeneration has occurred. However, diagnostic EMG is a very sensitive indicator of the physiological state of the muscle, which is directly affected by the functioning of the motor nerve axons. The AHC and motor nerve axons provide nutrients and stability to the muscle fibers they innervate. Proteins are provided via axoplasmic flow to the muscle, and when flow of these proteins is restricted or reduced, a decline in muscle stability occurs. Causes of muscle membrane instability include denervation, but also include compression, axonal degeneration, and spinal shock. Needle EMG allows evaluating a muscle membrane for instability by looking (and listening) for the sounds of abnormal waveforms that occur at rest.

This chapter will describe the type of normal and abnormal waveforms seen during a diagnostic EMG examination, and how this information is used to rule out or confirm a neurological diagnosis. If abnormalities are revealed in the EMG component of the exam, the neurological distribution of the muscles revealing abnormalities is extremely important. If a patient has a mononeuropathy, abnormalities on EMG would be isolated to one specific peripheral nerve distribution. In motor root compression (ex: radiculopathy at C5), the distribution of abnormalities should be common to the C5 root, but from muscles from at least two different peripheral nerves. The diagnostic process will be discussed in more detail later in this chapter and in the following chapter. The final diagnostic process is coupled with a history, clinical examination, the results of electroneuromyography testing, and other clinical and laboratory tests that when reviewed and analyzed in total, help to determine the pathological condition of the patient.

Nerve conduction testing and diagnostic EMG are within the practice act of physical therapists in almost every state. The objective of this book is not to instruct the reader to a depth of understanding and skill to be able to begin to perform this testing. The American Medical Association has stated support for Physical Therapist's who are qualified, to perform diagnostic EMG. This testing is an extension of a physical examination and evaluation and is very accurate in assisting the diagnosis of neuromuscular disorders.

Considerations for the insertion of needles, including a review of anatomy, universal precautions, and general technique are beyond the scope and intent of this publication.

Contraindications
- Blood clotting disorders
- Lymph node resections in that extremity.

- Lymphedema
- Immuno-compromised patients are at high risk for infection.

Precautions
- Indwelling cardiac pacemakers or deep brain stimulators or other indwelling devices
- Chest wall and abdominal muscle needle insertions
- Patients in ICU's, CCU's regarding intra-arterial catheters and proper electrical grounding.

Sampling and Recording Within the Muscle

The recording (needle) electrode is inserted into the belly of the muscle initially at a superficial level. The examiner looks (and listens) for electrical activity at rest and then asks the patient to lightly contract the muscle to obtain minimal MU recruitment. The muscle is evaluated by inserting the needle within the muscle at diagonals of 12, 3, 6, 9 o'clock, both superficially and deep.
- At each level of penetration, observe for electrical activity at rest and with minimal MU recruitment.
- At one level, test for complete interference pattern.

Needle Placement
- Motor Unit Territory – amplitude of the MUAP's in relation to the needle tip:
- .12 mm away from MU → 50% decrease in amplitude
- .38 mm away from MU → 90% decrease in amplitude

Normal EMG Waveforms at Rest
- Insertional activity – normal up to 300 ms after needle insertion. These waveforms are non-specific and cannot be individually identified. These waveforms occur when the needle electrode pierces the muscle membrane.
- Fasciculation potentials – these look like normal motor units, however their rate (frequency) of discharge is

irregular and they are not under voluntary control. If these are seen in one or two muscles, they are considered benign. They also occur in fatigue.
- Nerve Potential – touching an axon with the tip of the needle will result in seeing and hearing nerve potential.
- End Plate Noise – when the tip of needle is close to an end plate, the baseline will become elevated and it will sound like placing your ear to a conch shell. Miniature end plate potentials are normal and are due to small quanta of ACh being released into the NMJ.
- If a few normal motor units are seen "at rest", it means the muscle being tested is not fully relaxed.

Normal Motor Unit Action Potentials
- Duration = 7-12 ms
- Amplitude = 5 millivolts or less
- Phases = 2 – 4
- Frequency of firing (discharge) = regular
- They are under voluntary control!

Motor units are composed of the AHC, nerve axon and all the muscle fibers innervated by that AHC. The waveform produced by each depolarization is a summation of all the muscle fibers and is called a summated motor unit action potential (MUAP). Figure 6-1 represents three MU's, A, B & C. Motor unit "A" is composed of five muscle fibers. The action potential generated by each fiber is shown on the left and the summated MUAP is on the right. The amplitude is measured peak to peak of the summated MUAP, and the duration is the overall time in milliseconds of the entire summated MUAP. There are three phases in the summated MUAP below. Each phase is the number of waveforms above or below the baseline.

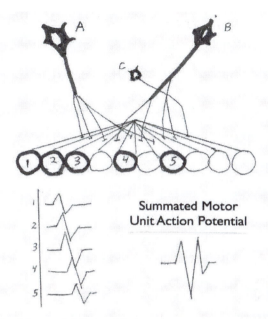

Figure 6-1: Normal Motor Unit

MU Recruitment and Interference Pattern

At very low levels of a normal muscle contraction, very few motor units are recruited. As force production requirements increase, the rate of firing of MU's increases, and additional motor units are recruited. This pattern of increased frequency of firing and additional MU's activated is called MU recruitment. If each individual motor unit action potential can be easily identified, with baseline between each motor unit, this is considered a single unit interference pattern. The top first and second horizontal tracings in Figure 6-2 represent a single unit interference pattern. There is some overlap of more than one motor unit firing, but there is baseline between each action potential (letters correspond to different MU's firing). This is normal at very low levels of a muscle contraction. However, if this is seen on maximal effort, there is a very serious loss of motor unit recruitment, which is typically indicative of severe axonal loss. The middle tracings represent an incomplete interference pattern.

There are more MU's firing, some MUAP's have merged visually due to simultaneous recruitment, but baseline is apparent in the tracing. This amount of motor unit recruitment is normal at a low level of effort, approximately equivalent to a 3 plus to 4 minus manual muscle testing grade. If this is the maximum recruitment an individual can produce in a specific muscle, there is a serious loss of motor units.

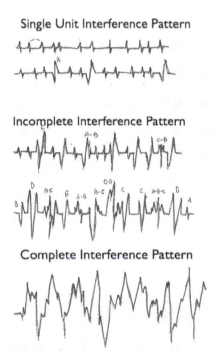

Figure 6-2: Motor Unit Recruitment Patterns

A complete interference pattern (CIP) on strong effort is a normal response (as seen in the bottom tracings). To achieve this level of MU recruitment only requires approximately 30% of maximum effort. A CIP does not indicate the muscle is fully innervated. Consider interpretation of an interference pattern as you would initially interpret manual muscle testing grades. Since a CIP requires only 30% of maximum motor unit recruitment, anything less than a CIP on maximal effort indicates significant loss of MU's. One exception is in patients with a myopathy. Due to reduced force production in each motor unit in this patient population, you will tend to see a CIP on early effort. This concept is extremely important in understanding overuse weakness in patients with a myopathy or polio. They recruit a greater percentage of motor units for typical ADL, and therefore have fewer motor units on reserve for prolonged or vigorous activities.

Summary of Interference Patterns (IP)
- Complete IP = should occur with strong effort in a healthy individual.
- Complete IP on early effort, with low amplitude – myopathy
- Incomplete IP on maximal effort = major loss of MU's, partial neuropathy
- Single Unit IP on maximal effort = severe loss of MU's and severe neuropathy

Pathological EMG Waveforms – At Rest
During diagnostic EMG, a normal muscle is electrically and physiologically stable. There are no biological potentials present and the term for this normal state is "silent at rest". Various biological potentials (ex: fibrillation potentials) that occur at rest are indicative of a disease process affecting the AHC, nerve axon, or muscle fibers. The muscle membranes become unstable resulting in pathological waveforms observed at rest during diagnostic EMG. The pathological waveforms at rest include:
- Increased insertional activity - prolonged, but unidentified electrical discharges after needle insertion or movement, indicative of muscle membrane instability. These findings are difficult to interpret if they are the only finding at rest along with normal motor units.

- <u>Fibrillation Potentials (Fibs)</u> - these are a specific type of electrical discharge at rest (Figure 6-3). They are most likely due to spontaneous discharges of individual muscle fibers. They are not a type of motor unit. They tend to fire at regular or irregular frequencies, and may sound like rain on a tin roof or crumbling paper. They are indicative of muscle membrane instability, usually the result of nerve damage or seen in a myopathy. Early literature considered these to be denervation potentials, however, they are also found in a patient during spinal shock, the flaccid state after a stroke, myopathy and other conditions.
- <u>Positive Sharp Waves</u> - these are another type of electrical discharge seen at rest (Figure 6-4). They are not a type of motor unit. They tend to fire at regular or irregular frequencies. Their waveform is downward on the screen and primarily one phase. They are also indicative of muscle membrane instability, which is usually the result of nerve damage or a myopathy.
- <u>Fasciculation Potentials</u> - these are the same as described at rest. They are irregular discharges of a motor unit, and not under voluntary control. They are diagnostically significant when seen in many muscles and are indicative of AHC or nerve axon instability or irritability.
- <u>High Frequency Discharges</u> - also called Myotonic discharges or bizarre discharges. They are prolonged, continuous electrical discharges at rest often seen in patients with different forms of myotonia. They are also found in patients with chronic myopathy, neuropathies, radiculopathy and AHC disease.

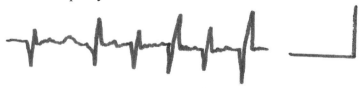

Figure 6-3: Fibrillation Potentials
Calibration = 100 uVolts vertical; 20 msec horizontal

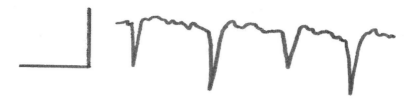

Figure 6-4: Positive Sharp Waves
Calibration = 100 uVolts vertical: 20 msec horizontal

Pathological Motor Units - Neuropathic Conditions
<u>Long Duration Motor Units</u>
- Duration = greater than 12 ms
- Amp = 2 millivolts or less
- Phases = 2 – 4
- Freq = regular

These motor units are longer in duration than normal motor units, but otherwise have normal characteristics. Motor units become longer in duration in the early stages of a demyelinating process. The timing of discharge of action potentials in each of the muscle fibers in the motor unit is more prolonged, and therefore the summation of all the muscle fibers discharging takes longer than normal. The slowing of the individual muscle fiber discharges also occurs in a myopathy. However, in a myopathy, motor units will also be decreasing in amplitude, which will be described later.

<u>Long Duration Polyphasic Motor Units</u>
- Duration = greater than 12 ms
- Amp = 2 millivolts or less
- Phases = 5 or more
- Freq = regular

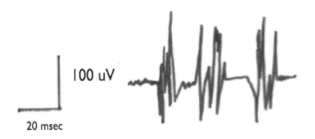

Figure 6-5: Long Duration Polyphasic Motor Units
Calibration = 100 uVolts vertical: 20 msec horizontal

Long Duration Polyphasic Motor Units (Figure 6-5) have multiple pathological electrical characteristics. The electrical conduction to each muscle fiber of the MU is more prolonged and some of the terminal end fibers of the axon have lost their ability to conduct an AP and activate the single muscle fiber it innervates. This results in a loss of contribution of some fibers to the summated MUAP and the electrical characteristics of each phase are more distorted. Multiple phases occur coupled with a prolonged duration from the discharge of the first muscle fiber to the last muscle fiber. Long Duration Polyphasic motor units are considered indicative of a neuropathy when more than 10% of the motor units observed in a muscle are polyphasic.

<u>Large Amplitude Motor Units</u>
- Duration = often long duration
- Amp = 5 millivolts & up
- Phases = often polyphasic
- Freq = regular

Large Amplitude motor units are seen as part of the healing process after a partial nerve injury. Denervated muscle fibers become sensitive to ACh along their entire muscle membrane, which serves as a chemical stimulant to trigger collateral sprouting from adjacent (intact) motor nerve axons. If collateral sprouting is successful, the intact motor unit will reinnervate these adjacent denervated muscle fibers. Therefore, the anatomical size of the intact motor unit has increased by adopting these new muscle fibers into its family. More muscle fibers contribute to a larger motor unit anatomically and electrically, resulting in a larger summated MUAP. The amplitude of the motor unit increases to larger than normal. This only occurs with collateral sprouting after a nerve injury, and more commonly occurs in a partial nerve injury. It takes a few months for large amplitude motor units to appear, therefore they are indicative of a prior, chronic nerve injury.

Pathological Motor Units - Myopathic Conditions
A patient with a myopathy has a disease affecting the stability of the muscle membrane, resulting in eventual muscle fiber necrosis. The peripheral nerves are essentially intact, and therefore conduction of motor axons is WNL. Pathological changes have been reported in the terminal branches of motor axons in the later stages of myopathy. Progression of the disease results in a loss of viable muscle fibers, and the person begins to loose strength in the affected muscles. In a myopathy, the loss of muscle fibers eventually results in a decrease in the amplitude and the overall duration of the motor unit action potential. These motor units may look like Fibrillation Potentials, however they are under voluntary control. Asking the patient to contract and then relax and seeing (hearing) the motor units appear and stop confirms that these are motor units under voluntary control and not fibrillation potentials, which are involuntary.

Short Duration Motor Units
- Duration = 1-5 ms
- Amp = 2 millivolts or less
- Phases = 2 – 4
- Freq = all MU are regular and under voluntary control.

Short duration motor units occur as a result of loss of muscle fibers within a motor unit. When the majority of fibers that contributes to the overall duration of the summated MUAP die off, this results in a motor unit that looks electrically shorter in duration than normal. This occurs only secondary to a myopathic process. EMG is one of the significant tests to rule in or rule out a myopathy based upon the electrical configuration of the motor units.

<u>Low Amplitude MU</u>
- Duration = 7 ms
- Amp = under 100 uV, often under 50 uV.
- Phases = 2 – 4
- Freq = all MU are regular and under voluntary control.

If muscle fibers contributing to the peak summation MUAP are affected first, the amplitude of these motor units will begin to fall below the normal range. In patients with a myopathy, eventually motor units increasingly become short duration and low amplitude compared to normal. Therefore, the typical finding in someone with a myopathy is a majority of motor units being low amplitude, short duration. An examination that reveals these myopathic motor units helps confirm a myopathy, but does not assist in determining the type of myopathy the individual has. However, low amplitude, long duration polyphasic MU's are also found in some myopathic conditions. The ultimate diagnosis is a combination of a comprehensive history and evaluation that may include a PT, neurologist, blood chemistry, genetic testing and muscle biopsy.

Figure 6-6 displays short duration, low amplitude motor units, which is a combination of the two typical changes associated with a myopathic process.

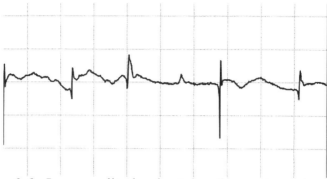

Figure 6-6: Low amplitude, short duration motor units
Calibration settings 100uv vertically; 10 ms horizontally.
Photograph used with permission: Cadwell Laboratories, Inc.

Summary and Review
Standard motor conduction studies and SNAP's evaluate the peripheral nervous system for deficits in conduction of action potentials along segments of the peripheral nervous system. The findings contribute to the overall evaluation of the patient to determine if and where a pathological process may be present.

Advanced conduction techniques evaluate the function of the proximal segments of the peripheral nervous system and central nervous system tracts regarding ability to conduct an AP.

During diagnostic EMG – abnormalities at rest indicate instability of muscle membranes, which occur with nerve or muscle disorders. The types of motor units seen are a key factor in differentiating a neuropathic process from a myopathic process. Coupled with the clinical findings clinicians can often diagnosis the type of a neuromuscular disorders. The distribution and pattern of findings during diagnostic EMG help reveal the location and type of disorder.

Motor units are either:
Myopathic - Short Duration and/or Low Amplitude
Normal - Normal Duration and Normal Amplitude
Neuropathic – Long Duration, Long Duration Polyphasic and/or Large Amplitude.

Selection of Appropriate Muscles for Testing
- Based upon history, initial evaluation, results of performing SNAP's and MCV's. What do you need to know next to help determine diagnosis and severity?
- If first muscle tested reveals abnormalities, what needs to be tested next to a reveal a pattern of pathology that supports a diagnosis?
- What other NCV/EMG tests should be performed to rule out other pathological conditions?
- If testing reveals no abnormalities, how should the clinician proceed with his/her evaluation of the patient?

These concepts/questions will be reviewed in Chapter seven.

CHAPTER SEVEN

Problem Solving in Electroneuromyography and Case Studies

This chapter will review the critical thinking and problem-solving approach used in electrophysiologic testing and physical therapy evaluative procedures that are used collaboratively to clarify the diagnosis of the patients with disorders of the neuromuscular system.

The decision making process in physical therapy examination is threaded throughout most physical therapy curricula. The first section of this chapter should be a review of what the physical therapy student or clinician has previously learned and developed a level of competency. This is a summary of a screening assessment and decision-making process used during an evaluation of a patient to determine what area of the neuromuscular system requires more specific attention.

Observation of the Patient
The evaluation of a patient begins with your first greeting and interaction while observing how the patient gets up from a chair in the waiting room, ambulates to the examination room, and prepares for your interview and examination. Note any of the following before you ask your first question.
- Obvious guarding, weakness, atrophy, gait deviations, asymmetry.
- How does the patient present for examination? Are movement patterns irregularly, inconsistently, require your assistance. Is the patient using an orthotic or assistive device?

History of the Patient
What brings the patient in for this evaluation? What are their primary complaints, symptoms and difficulties in ADL?
Past medical history may give some insight into their current condition, including a listing of all medications the patient is currently taking or required in the past. PMH of cancer and chemotherapy agents, diabetes medications, etc. all provides significant insight to the potential current problems.

- Past medical history
- Chief complaints?
- Complaints - are they continuous or sporadic ex: worse at night, worse with activity, changes with rest.
- Onset of symptoms - abrupt or slow?
- Signs and symptoms - localized - unilateral or generalized?
- Proximal or distal?
- Bilateral, symmetrical or irregular?
- How long have these symptoms/complaints been present?
- Does patient associate problem with a specific injury?
- Prior evaluations/tests? What were the results?
- What does patient think the cause of the problem is?
- Do other family members have similar problems?

Physical Examination
Skin
- Color & temperature
  - Neurogenic - color & temperature is normal
  - Vascular - blue due to venous insufficiency and pale is due to arterial insufficiency. Limb segment is cold.
- Trophic Changes
  - Neurogenic - skin is dry due to denervation of sweat glands.
  - Vascular - hair loss, shiny skin.

Motor
- Atrophy
- Hypertrophy/Pseudohypertrophy
- Spasticity/Rigidity
- Fasciculation's
- Muscle testing results

Sensory
- Numbness, decreased sensation - hypoesthesia
- Pins & needles, tingling - paresthesia (large fiber involvement)
- Burning - dysesthia (small fiber involvement).
- Increased sensitivity – hyperesthesia
- Vibration - intact distally?
- Joint Position Sense - intact distally?

Deep Tendon Reflexes
- Absent
- Normal
- Hyper-reflexive

Assessment – Did the findings reveal?
- Normal Assessment
- Unilateral involvement
- Sensory abnormalities
    - in a peripheral nerve distribution?
    - in a root distribution?
    - present in multiple peripheral nerves or root distributions?
    - revealing CNS signs (ex: graphesthesia, stereognosis)
- Motor abnormalities
    - in a peripheral nerve distribution?
    - in a root distribution?
    - present in multiple peripheral nerves or root distributions?
    - revealing CNS signs

- Combinations of more than one of the above
- Bilateral or all four extremities involvement
  - Sensory
  - Motor
  - Symmetrical or asymmetrical in BUE's or BLE's.
  - Significance of Proximal vs. Distal findings

Review – In suspected peripheral nerve involvement
What nerve conduction studies would you perform?
What muscles would you select for electromyography?

Review – In suspected root involvement
What nerve conduction studies would you perform?
What muscles would you select for electromyography?

The following thirteen case studies are progressively designed to test and guide the reader in determining how nerve conductions studies, diagnostic EMG, and other advanced techniques can assist in determining the diagnosis of a patient. The answers for each case study immediately follow. Proceed through these examples, referring back to the prior sections as needed to best answer the questions. In the first set of cases, determine what you might expect the results to reveal if you referred a patient for testing and you were correct in your preliminary diagnosis. Patient clinical descriptions and presentations are brief to provide general information.

Case Study # 1: Carpal Tunnel Syndrome
Minimal atrophy of the APB, clumsiness & sensory loss.

Describe the findings of:
SNAP's.
NCV's-
EMG-

Answers:
- Median nerve SNAP's would reveal a prolonged latency. Amplitude would be decreased. The SNAP might even be absent if the compression has progressed to causing muscle atrophy which is associated with more severe nerve compression and axonal degeneration. Median nerve motor nerve conduction velocity in the forearm would be normal.
- Ulnar SNAP's should have been performed and should be normal (ulnar nerve is external to the carpal tunnel).
- The opposite hand should have all of the above tests performed. Often CTS is bilateral, even with only unilateral symptoms.
- EMG of the APB would reveal fibrillation potentials and positive sharp waves at rest. Motor units would include normal, plus long duration polyphasic motor units. Interference pattern should be complete unless atrophy and motor nerve compression has moderately occurred with associated conduction block and/or axonal loss.
- Literature also supports a double crush syndrome in which may patients with CTS also have root compression. Depending upon symptoms, testing for cervical root compression may be appropriate. Patients with diabetes are also more at risk for developing CTS.

Case Study # 2: Age 5 – Duchenne MD (DMD)

How would patient present? Describe the findings of:
SNAP's.
NCV's-
EMG-

Answer:
- A boy with suspected DMD would present with a positive Gower's maneuver, ambulate on his toes, have an increased lumbar lordosis, and proximal weakness in

his UE's and LE's. If laboratory testing has not been done, an EMG should not be done prior to drawing blood for CPK and other testing.
- SNAP testing, if performed, should all be WNL's. One UE and one LE nerve might be tested.
- Motor nerve conduction studies should all be WNL's. The amplitude of the CMAP with MCV's may be decreased.
- EMG testing may reveal abnormalities at rest in proximal vs. distal muscles tested. These may include fibrillation potentials and/or positive sharp waves in more severely involved proximal muscles.
- The most significant finding to confirm a diagnosis of DMD would be short duration and/or low amplitude motor units in many, if not all of the muscles examined. Testing should be at a minimum. Motor unit recruitment may reveal a complete interference pattern on early effort. This occurs because as the muscle force production declines in muscular dystrophy, the patient must recruit many more motor units to produce adequate force production for movement or functional activities.
- This is strictly a summary for this diagnostic category.

Case Study # 3: Suspected L5 Root Compression

How would patient present? Describe the findings of:
SNAP's.
NCV's-
EMG-

Answer:
- Patient will report sensory complaints in the distribution if a sensory root being compressed.
- There may also be motor weakness in the root distribution if the motor root is being compressed. This requires more severe compression to be obvious on

manual muscle testing, with weakness in the distribution of the root involved. Ex: anterior tibialis, fibularis longus, fibularis brevis, and/or extensor hallucis longus.
- SNAP's should all be WNL's.
- Motor conduction studies should also be all WNL's. If there is severe motor axonal damage, then the amplitude of the CMAP's will begin to decrease.
- H-reflex and/or F-wave testing would be normal if performed using the gastrocnemius muscle, which is considered to be primarily innervated by S1.
- EMG testing would reveal abnormalities at rest in muscles innervated by the involved root segment. A gold standard that helps confirm involvement at the root level is finding EMG abnormalities at rest in the paravertebral muscles innervated by the involved motor root.

Confirming Root Compression – How do you rule in or rule out root compression compared to (for example) Piriformis Syndrome? The diagram in Figure 7-1 shows a cross section of the spinal cord, the pathways of the posterior and anterior roots, and how these roots join prior to exiting the intervertebral foramen. After exiting, the combined root splits into the anterior and posterior primary rami. The significance of these pathways is that the anterior primary rami form the peripheral nerves to the extremities, and the posterior primary rami exit and innervate the paravertebral muscles. The EMG abnormalities at rest (fibrillation potentials and/or positive sharp waves) in the paravertebral muscles are indicative of root compression. Involvement distal to the intervertebral foramen (such as piriformis syndrome) would result in abnormalities in the extremity muscles but the paravertebral muscles would be normal.

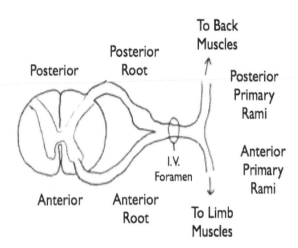

Figure 7-1: Formation of Anterior and Posterior Primary Rami

Case Study # 4: Suspected Peripheral Polyneuropathy
May be seen in patients with diabetes, alcohol abuse, heavy metal or drug toxicity, hereditary motor & sensory neuropathy (Charcot-Marie-Tooth disease), Guillian-Barre' Syndrome, etc.

How would patient present? Describe the findings of:
SNAP's.
NCV's-
EMG-

Answer:
- Many peripheral neuropathies present the same, but the etiology is varied.
- The patient presents with sensory complaints in a glove and stocking distribution prior to the onset of significant motor complaints. Distal LE's symptoms occur prior to UE symptoms, but a proximal neuropathy may manifest first. An example of a proximal neuropathy is a femoral neuropathy presenting as isolated quadriceps weakness.

- Deep tendon reflexes will be reduced or absent, also distally prior to proximally.
- SNAP's reveal the first abnormality. SNAP's of the LE may reveal decreased amplitude prior to prolonged latency. Specialized testing of the Medial Plantar and Dorsal Sural nerve has been reported to increase the sensitivity in diagnosing early stage peripheral neuropathies.
- Nerve conduction velocities will be decreased in demyelinating peripheral neuropathies.
- Amplitude of SNAP's will be decreased in axonal degeneration.
- EMG changes will evolve when motor axons are more involved. Abnormalities at rest may be present, coupled with long duration motor units and/or long duration polyphasic motor units. Large amplitude motor units are indicative of a chronic neuropathy where regeneration and/or reinnervation have also occurred.
- Interference pattern should be complete except in severe cases of progressive polyneuropathy.

Case Study #5: EMG Report #1
What do the findings reveal and what might the diagnosis be, prior to knowing the history and physical examination?

Motor Conduction Right		Latency (msec)	CV (m/sec)
Median	Wrist→APB	2.5 (Nml)	El→Wr 64.6 (Nml)
Ulnar	Wrist→ADM	2.1 (Nml)	El→Wr 67.0 (Nml)
Fibular	Ankle→EDB	3.2 (Nml)	Kn→An 52.4 (Nml)

SNAP's Right		Latency (msec)	Amplitude (uV)
Median	Wrist→ II	2.0 (Nml)	54 (Nml)
Ulnar	Wrist→ V	1.8 (Nml)	59 (Nml)
Superf. Fib.	Calf→Ankle	2.1 (Nml)	26 (Nml)

Electromyography	Findings
Right Biceps Right ABP Right 1st DI Right Vastus M. Right Ant. Tib.	Silent at rest. Normal, short duration and low amplitude motor units on volition with complete interference pattern (CIP) on early effort.
Right & Left Deltoid	Fibrillation potentials at rest. Normal and short duration polyphasic motor units on volition with a complete interference pattern on early effort.

Analysis and Answer:
- Motor and sensory nerve conduction studies are all WNL's. This helps rule out peripheral nerve involvement.
- EMG findings at rest are often normal in someone with an early clinical picture. Later, as the disease progresses, abnormalities are often found at rest. In the late stages of the disease (although the diagnosis should have been made long ago), there may not be any abnormalities at rest.
- The finding of short duration types of motor units is highly suggestive of a myopathy and the most significant finding in this report. Low amplitude motor units are also found in this patient population.
- A complete interference pattern on early effort is suggestive of more muscle fiber loss in this specific muscle.
- These findings are classical in a patient with a myopathy. The diagnosis is made or ruled out using EMG, clinical findings, laboratory tests (CPK blood enzymes), genetic testing and muscle biopsy as deemed necessary.

Case Study #6: EMG Report #2
What do the findings reveal and what is a possible diagnosis?

Motor Conduction   Latency (msec)   CV (m/sec)
Right
Median Wrist→APB   3.3 (Nml)   El→Wr 54.4 (Nml)
Ulnar   Wrist→ADM   3.1 (Nml)   El→Wr 57.2 (Nml)
Fibular Ankle→EDB   3.7 (Nml)   Kn→An 50.4 (Nml)

SNAP's   Latency (msec)   Amplitude (uV)
Right
Median Wrist→ II   2.3 (Nml)   84 (Nml)
Ulnar Wrist→ V   2.1 (Nml)   62 (Nml)
Superf. Fib. Calf→Ankle   2.7 (Nml)   19 (Nml)

Electromyography	Findings
Right Deltoid	Increased insertion activity, fibrillation potentials, positive sharp waves, and fasciculation potentials at rest. Normal, large amplitude and polyphasic motor units potentials on volition. CIP on strong effort.
Right ABP	
Right 1st DI	
Right Biceps B.	
Right Triceps B.	
Right FCR	
Left Deltoid	
Left FCR	
Right & Left Vastus M.	
Right & Left Anterior Tib.	
Right & Left Upper Trapezius	Increased insertion activity, fibrillation potentials and fasciculation potentials at rest. Long duration polyphasic motor units on volition.

Patient history:
Forty-year-old male with atrophy and weakness of both hands for the past eight months. He reports progressive muscle twitching in all four extremities with occasional muscle cramps in both hands. He has a history of swallowing problems for the past two years. Reflexes are all hyperactive; sensation is WNL's throughout all four extremities.

Answer to #6:
- Motor and sensory nerve conduction studies are all WNL's. This helps rule out peripheral nerve involvement.
- There are abnormalities at rest in many muscles of the upper and lower extremities. Findings are bilateral, with less sampling of muscles on the left side but more comprehensive sampling of muscles on the right. Note that findings are similar in proximal or distal muscles, in the upper or lower extremity.
- There are large amplitude and long duration polyphasic motor units in almost all muscles. Large amplitude motor units are indicative of a chronic condition with some re-innervation and long duration polyphasic motor units are indicative of a neuropathic process.
- Testing of the upper trapezius muscle bilaterally reveals less significant abnormalities, but supports cranial nerve involvement coupled with a systemic motor involvement.
- These findings, coupled with the history described above, are indicative of a diagnosis of chronic, progressive motor neuron disease, such as ALS.
- More specific diagnostic assessment is required to confirm this diagnosis (ex: El Escorial guidelines).

Case Study #7: EMG Report #3
What do the findings reveal and what do you feel the diagnosis might be? What other testing might you add and

what would the results need to be to help confirm your diagnosis?

<u>Motor Conduction</u> Latency (msec)   <u>CV</u> (m/sec)
Right
Fibular   Ankle→EDB 4.7 (Nml)   Kn→An 48.4 (Nml)

<u>SNAP's</u>   Latency (msec)   Amplitude (uV)
Right
Sural   Calf→Ankle 3.3 (Nml)   20 (Nml)
Superf. Fib. Calf→Ankle 2.7 (Nml)   19 (Nml)

<u>Electromyography</u>	Findings
Right Anterior Tibialis Right Tensor Fascia Lata	Increased insertion activity, fibrillation potentials and positive sharp waves at rest. Normal and polyphasic motor units potentials on volition. CIP on strong effort.
Right paravertebrals L4-5	High frequency discharges and fibrillation potentials at rest. Normal and long duration polyphasic motor unit potentials on volition.
Right Extensor Hallus Longus	Increased insertion activity at rest. Normal motor units on volition.
Right paravertebrals L3-L5 Right fibularis longus Right vastus medialis Right gastrocnemius	Silent at rest. Normal motor units on volition.

Answer:
- Motor and sensory conduction studies are all WNL's.
- EMG findings reveal abnormalities at rest in the right anterior tibialis (L4-5, fibular nerve), tensor fascia lata (L4-S1, superior gluteal nerve) and paravertebrally alongside L4-5. Abnormalities in muscles from more than one peripheral nerve but with the same nerve root(s) in common is classic for a diagnosis of root compression. The additional findings of abnormalities at rest in the paravertebral muscles alongside the same spinal level are the gold standard for confirming the diagnosis of L4-5 root compression.
- Testing that may help confirm root compression include a F-wave. Results may include lower amplitude and/or prolonged latency and combined with EMG results support motor root compression.
- The diagnosis of a L4-5 radiculopathy only indicates what nerve root is involved, but does not anatomically locate the site of the compression. A posterior-lateral disc herniation at L2 or L3 could also compress the L4 or L5 root as it passes caudally in the spinal canal.

Case Study #8: Gun Shot Wound to the Cauda Equina, L1 - L2.

This is an example of using NCV's and EMG to determine current state of recovery and prognosis for future recovery.

Motor Conduction		Latency (msec)
Right		
Fibular	Fibula head→Anterior Tibialis	5.1
	Popliteal fossa→Fibularis Longus	4.6
Tibial	Popliteal fossa→Med Gastroc.	4.8

SNAP's	Latency (msec)	Amplitude (uV)
Right		
Sural	Calf→Ankle 2.5 (Nml)	8.0 (Low)

Superf. Fib.	Leg→Ankle	2.0 (Nml)	5.0 (Low)
Left Sural	Calf→Ankle	2.4 (Nml)	10.0 (Low)

Electromyography	Findings
Right & Left Anterior Tibialis	Increased insertion activity, fibrillation potentials and positive sharp waves at rest. Few long duration polyphasic motor units potentials on volition. Single unit interference pattern on strong effort.
Right Med. Gastroc. Right tensor fascia lata Right & Left Gluteus Max Right Anal Sphincter	Increased insertion activity, fibrillation potentials and positive sharp waves at rest. No motor units on volition.

Explanation of the testing:
- Stimulating any motor nerve and recording a latency to one or more muscles innervated by that peripheral nerve confirm the muscle is innervated. This is more meaningful than "is this latency WNL's"?

What does this tell the physician and therapists?
- The anterior tibialis and fibularis longus on the right, plus the left medial gastrocnemius are all partially innervated.
- The sensory nerves listed are all conducting. The low amplitude indicates additional regeneration of axons may still be occurring, but sensory innervation is present. The initial lesion may be proximal to the dorsal root ganglia.
- EMG findings are important for those muscles with motor units found on voluntary contraction. A single unit interference pattern is the earliest sign of motor axon regeneration and reinnervation, with the neuromuscular

junction stabile enough to produce a consistently firing motor unit. With time, there is the possibility of additional motor nerve axons regenerating and reinnervating some of the remaining muscle fibers. Interference pattern may become incomplete with the formation of additional MU's.
- Muscles listed with fibrillation potential and positive sharp waves are confirming these muscles are denervated, but that there is also viable muscle tissue present. Reinnervation is still possible.
- Testing the anal sphincter is one method of determining if sacral reinnervation is occurring.

Case Studies 9 - 13:
Determine the least amount of testing and the results for each of the following. For any acute injury, testing must be delayed at least 14 days:

Case #9: Anterior Glenohumeral Joint Dislocation

Case #10: Mid Humeral Fracture

Case #11: Multiple Sclerosis

Case #12: Isolated Scapula Winging

Case #13: Idiopathic Bell's Palsy

Answers to Group Three:

Case #9: Anterior Glenohumeral Joint Dislocation
The diagnosis of axillary nerve damage is often not investigated in the acute management of this injury. After therapy begins, the patient may present with severe "weakness" of the deltoid. EMG of the deltoid would help determine if a traction injury occurred to the axillary nerve

during the dislocation. The testing must not be performed until at least two weeks after the injury (see chapter one). Fibrillation potentials and/or positive sharp waves would be indicative of nerve damage. Motor units may be long duration polyphasic or absent if a complete nerve injury occurred. Interference pattern would help reveal the severity of the nerve damage. Anything less than a complete interference pattern would reveal severe nerve damage.

Sensory disturbances would be limited to an area over the middle deltoid. EMG testing of the biceps brachii, supraspinatus and/or other muscles would be performed as indicated if there was any possibility of other peripheral nerve or brachial plexus involvement.

Case #10: Mid Humeral Fracture
Same basic approach as above, but the testing now is for the radial nerve. The radial nerve pathway includes the radial groove, and mid-humeral displaced fractures can result in immediate injury, while delayed injury of the radial nerve can occur due to entrapment of the radial nerve in the callous formation at the fracture site. The triceps is mostly unaffected, but the medial head of the triceps and distally innervated muscles of the radial nerve may be affected.

EMG abnormalities may be found in all other radial nerve innervated muscles in the forearm, including the brachioradialis. Severe injury results in wrist drop and paralysis of the finger extensors. Anything less than a complete interference pattern would reveal severe nerve damage.

Case #11: Multiple Sclerosis
Electrophysiologic testing is not indicated in this patient, unless concurrent peripheral involvement is suspected. All peripheral nerve testing should be WNL's.

Somatosensory evoked potentials might be abnormal if the sensory tracts of the spinal cord are affected. However, SSEP's are not the primary diagnostic test for MS.

This diagnosis is listed here strictly to remind the reader that MS is a CNS disorder and the testing in this publication is not typically performed.

Case #12: Isolated Scapula Winging
The long thoracic nerve innervates the serratus anterior. There is no sensory distribution to this nerve, so symptoms are limited and mild weakness may be overlooked. Nerve injury would manifest as asymmetrical scapula winging and inability to actively and fully flex the arm to 180 degrees. Involvement is isolated to the serratus anterior and EMG would reveal abnormalities at rest and long duration polyphasic motor units. Injury can be due to carrying a heavy shoulder bag, post mastectomy or upper extremity and scapula movements of high velocity and large excursions.

Case #13: Idiopathic Bell's Palsy
EMG testing of facial muscles will reveal abnormalities at rest. Testing should include a sampling of muscles in each branch of the facial nerve. After performing needle EMG examination, a latency value can be determined by leaving the needle inserted and stimulating the facial nerve anterior to the external auditory meatus. This would help determine the conductivity of the specific branch of the facial nerve to confirm if a proximal neurapraxia is producing the weakness or if there is more severe axonal degeneration. Muscles tested should minimally include the frontalis, orbicularis oculi and the orbicularis oris. Isolated lesions to a branch of the facial nerve may occur secondary to surgery or trauma, which is different than idiopathic Bell's Palsy.

Appendix A

Anatomical Correlates and Associated Impairments

Sensory Neurons - decreased or absent sensory awareness including one or more of the following: light touch, pain, temperature, proprioception and/or vibration.

Myopathy - weakness in proximal muscle groups before more distal involvement. Distribution of weakness varies in different forms of myopathy. Steroid myopathy, polymyositis and other myopathies will also present with proximal weakness and similar electrodiagnostic results.

Neuromuscular Junction - undue fatigue that progresses with activity. Worsens as the day progresses, improves with rest.

Anterior Horn Cell - as in polio, ALS, Spinal Muscular Atrophy. Weakness or flaccid paralysis in all AHC diseases, with associated UMN signs in ALS.

Spinal Cord Injury - UMN signs, weakness or flaccidity below the injury. Possible LMN signs at the level of injury.

Cerebellum* - incoordination, possible deconditioning and impaired aerobic capacity. Balance deficits.

Basal Ganglia* - bradykinesia or absence of movement. Rigidity and tremor at rest. Significant movement impairment as the disease progresses.

Motor & Premotor Cortex* - Paralysis, weakness or impairment of motor planning/execution.

Sensory Cortex* - loss or deficits of cortical sensations: Two point discrimination; graphesthesia; stereognosis; localization; bilateral simultaneous discrimination.

* Strictly a CNS disorder and electroneuromyography is not indicated.

Appendix B

Common Causes of Peripheral Neuropathies

Mononeuropathy

- Compression
- Diabetes
- Herpes Zoster
- Trauma
- Tumor
- Infectious processes
- Trigeminal Neuralgia
- Ischemia

Mononeuropathy Multiplex
- Multiple compression
- Diabetes
- Infectious processes
- Malignancy

Polyneuropathy
- Diabetes
- Kidney disease
- Lyme disease
- Alcoholic neuropathy
- Anti-viral medications ex HIV/AIDS
- Chemotherapy meds ex: Vincristine
- High Blood pressure meds
- Nutritional deficiencies, Vitamin B
- Guillian Barre' Syndrome
- Heavy Metals - Lead, Mercury
- Charcot-Marie-Tooth Disease (Hereditary Motor Sensory Neuropathy I).

Appendix C

Upper Extremity - Root and Peripheral Nerve Innervations

C 5-6	Deltoid (axillary nerve)
C 5-6	Biceps Brachii (musculocutaneous)
C 5-6	Brachioradialis (radial)
C 5-6	Supraspinatus (suprascapular)
C 7-8	Triceps (radial)
C 6-7	Extensor carpi radialis l & b (radial)
C 6, 7	Flexor carpi radialis (median)
C 7-8, T1	Flexor carpi ulnaris (ulnar)
C 8, T1	Abductor pollicis brevis (median)
C 8, T1	Abductor digiti minimi (ulnar)
C 8, T1	First dorsal interossei (ulnar)

(LE continued on next page)

Lower Extremity - Root and Peripheral Nerve Innervations

L 2, 3, 4	Quadriceps femoris (femoral nerve
L 4-5	Anterior tibialis (common fibular)
L 5, S1	Fibularis longus (common fibular)
L 4-5, S1	Tensor fascia lata (superior gluteal nerve)
L 5, S1-2	Gluteus maximus ((inferior gluteal nerve)
L 5, S1-2	Biceps femoris - short head (Sciatic-fib div)
L 5, S1-2	Biceps femoris - long head (Sciatic-tibial div)
L 5 - S1	Extensor hallucis longus (deep fibular)
S 1 - S2	Gastrocnemius (tibial)
L 5, S1-S2	Soleus (tibial)

References

Agur, A. M. R. & Dalley, A. F. (2013). *Grant's Atlas of Anatomy*. (13th ed.). Philadelphia, PA: Wolters Kluwer - Lippincott Williams & Wilkins.

Akuthota V, Plastaras C, Lindberg K, Tobey J, Press J, & Garvan C. The effect of long-distance bicycling on ulnar and median nerves: An electrophysiologic evaluation of cyclist palsy. Am J of Sports Med 2005; 33(8):1224-1230.

American Physical Therapy Association. (2001). Guide to Physical Therapist Practice. (2nd ed.). *Physical Therapy*. 81, 9-744.

Babyar, S. R. & Krasilovsky, G. (2006). Musculoskeletal Pattern 4C: Muscle Performance. In: M. Moffat and E. Rosen, (Eds), (2006) *Musculoskeletal Essentials: Applying the Physical Therapists Preferred Practice Patterns*, Thorofare, NJ: Slack Inc.

Echternach, J. L. (2003). *Introduction to Electromyography and Nerve Conduction Testing*. (2nd ed.). Thorofare, NJ: Slack Inc.

Braune, H. J. & Wunderlich, M. T. (1997). Diagnostic Value of Different Neurophysiological Methods in the Assessment of Lumbar Nerve Root Lesions, *Archives of Physical Medicine & Rehabilitation*, 78, 518-520.

DeLisa JA, Lee HJ, Baran EM, et al. (1994). *Manual of nerve conduction velocity and clinical neurophysiology*. (3rd ed). Baltimore: Lippincott Williams & Wilkins.

Goodgold, J. & Eberstein, A. (1983). *Electrodiagnosis of Neuromuscular Diseases.* (3rd ed.). Baltimore, MD; Williams and Wilkins.

Kennedy J. Neurologic injuries in cycling and bike riding. Neurol Clinics 2008;26(1):271-279.

Kim, C. T. et al., (2005). Neuromuscular Rehabilitation and Electrodiagnosis. 4. Pediatric Issues. *Archives of Physical Medicine & Rehabilitation*, 86(3 Suppl 1), S28-32.

Kimura, J. (2001). *Electrodiagnosis in Diseases of Nerve and Muscle: Principles and Practice.* (3rd ed.). Philadelphia, PA: F.A. Davis.

Krasilovsky, G. (1980). Nerve Conduction Studies in Patients with Cervical Spinal Cord Injury. *Archives of Physical Medicine & Rehabilitation,* 61, 204-209.

Mehreteab, T. A., Krasilovsky, G., Sandvik, S., Kuehn, L. & Gallentine, A. (2008). Impaired Peripheral Nerve Integrity and Muscle Performance Associated with Peripheral Nerve Injury (Pattern F). In: M. Moffat, J. Bohmert, J. B. Hulme (Eds), *Neuromuscular Essentials: Applying the Preferred Physical Therapist Practice Pattern*, Thorofare, NJ: Slack Inc.

NIOSH. *Performing Motor and Sensory Neuronal Conduction Studies in Adult Humans.* (1990). U.S Department of Health and Human Services, National Institute for Occupational Safety and Health, Washington, DC.

Oh, S. J. (1988). *Electromyography. Neuromuscular Transmission Studies*. Baltimore, MD: Williams & Wilkins.

O'Sullivan, S. O. & Schmitz, T. J. (2007). *Physical Rehabilitation: Assessment and Treatment.* (5th ed.). Philadelphia, PA: FA Davis.

Rayan, G. (1997). *Compression Neuropathies, Including Carpal Tunnel Syndrome.* Clinical Symposia, Vol. 39, 2, Novartis.

Robinson, A. J. (2008). Clinical Electrophysiologic Examination and Evaluation: Principles, Procedures, and Interpretation of Findings. In: A. J. Robinson & L. Synder-Mackler. *Clinical Electrophysiology. Electrotherapy and Electrophysiologic Testing,* Philadelphia, PA: Wolters Kluwer - Lippincott Williams & Wilkins.

Seddon, H. (1975). *Surgical Disorders of the Peripheral Nerves.* 2nd ed.) Edinburgh, Churchill Livingstone.

Strommen, J. A, et al., (2005). Neuromuscular Rehabilitation and Electrodiagnosis. 3. Diseases of Muscles and Neuromuscular Function. *Archives of Physical Medicine & Rehabilitation,* 86(3 Suppl 1), S18-27.

Sunderland, S. (1978). *Nerve and Nerve Injuries.* (2nd ed.) Edinburgh, Churchill Livingstone.

Troger, M, and Dengler R. (2000). The role of electromyography (EMG) in the diagnosis of ALS. *ALS,* supplement 2, 33-40.

Uluc, K., Isak, B., Borucu, D., et al. (2008). Medial plantar and dorsal sural nerve conduction studies increase the sensitivity in the detection of neuropathy in diabetic patients. *Clinical Neurophysiology,* 119, 880-885.

Upton AR, McComas AJ. (1973). The double crush in nerve

entrapment syndromes. *Lancet*; 2(7825), 359–62.

Visser, C. P. L., Tavy, D. L. J., Coene, L. and Brand, R. (1999). Electromyographic findings in shoulder dislocations and fractures of the proximal humerus: comparison with clinical neurological examination. *Clinical Neurology and Neurosurgery,* 101, 86-91.

Walsworth, M. K., Mills, J. T. & Michener, L. A. (2004). Diagnosing Suprascapular Neuropathy in Patients with Shoulder Dysfunction: A Report of 5 Cases. *Physical Therapy*, 84, 359-372.

Watson, L. A., Pizzari, T. & Balster, S. (2009). Thoracic outlet syndrome part 1: Clinical manifestations, differentiation and treatment pathways. *Manual Therapy*, 14, 586-595.

Watson, L. A., Pizzari, T. & Balster, S. (2010). Thoracic outlet syndrome part 2: Conservative Management. *Manual Therapy*, 15, 305-314.

Weiss, L. D., et al., (2005). Neuromuscular Rehabilitation and Electrodiagnosis. 2. Peripheral Neuropathy. *Archives of Physical Medicine & Rehabilitation*, 86 (3 Suppl 1), S11-7.

Williams, F. H., et al, (2005). Neuromuscular Rehabilitation and Electrodiagnosis. 1. Mononeuropathy. *Archives of Physical Medicine & Rehabilitation,* 86, (Suppl 1), S3-10.

Notes

Notes

Made in the USA
Charleston, SC
02 June 2015